THE 8 LOST ANCIENT SECRETS

TO BAKING SOURDOUGH BREAD

> *Unlocking the secrets to the original ancestral sourdough bread baking recipe.*

Let's put the record straight so there can be no more confusion. Real leavened bread, as made by our ancestors for thousands of years, was made with 3 ingredients.

1: 100% freshly milled organic whole grain wheat flour
2: Filtered water.
3: Natural grey sea salt. (Celtic sea salt is the only salt to be scientifically validated to contain 84 minerals)

Nothing removed from the flour, (The bran, germ, and starch remain intact).
Nothing added, by that I mean, dough conditioners, flour improvers, processing aids, chemical leavening, or any other artificial additives.

Food 4 Families Project
Clontarf, Queensland, 4019
Australia

MEDICAL DISCLAIMER

This content is for informational and educational purposes only. It is not intended to provide medical advice or to take the place of such advice or treatment from a personal physician. All readers/viewers of this content are advised to consult their doctor, or qualified health professionals, regarding specific health questions. Neither Peter McDonald, nor the publisher of this content takes responsibility for possible health consequences, of any person, or persons reading or following the information in this educational content. All viewers of this content, especially those taking prescription, or over-the-counter medications, should consult their physicians before beginning any nutrition, supplement, or lifestyle program.

Ordering Information:

For details, contact ganopeter@yahoo.com.au
www.food4familiesproject.com

Printed in Australia

CONTENTS

ACKNOWLEDGEMENTS

To the greatest gift I have been given

The Father, the Son, and the Holy Spirit

My Lord, my God, and my King

All the glory and honor go to You.

To my wonderful family, my wife, Alma,

And children, Chloe, John-Paul,

Nicole, Simon, and Benjamin

You are my inspiration,

And I thank you for the joy and happiness

You bring to my life.

It has been an amazing journey.

To my very talented and humble niece, Rhea Mae Alibong

For your great work on editing and laying out this book.

INTRODUCTION

"HOW COULD WHEAT AND GLUTEN, PRESENT IN A STAPLE FOOD LIKE BREAD, THAT HAS SUSTAINED HUMANITY FOR THOUSANDS OF YEARS, SUDDENLY BECOME THE BAD GUYS?" IT DEFIES LOGIC

Truth is, there's a lot of contradictory and even outright false information floating around about "REAL BREAD". That's why this book was written, because of all the misinformation, about the so-called, detrimental effect bread has on our health, it's a fallacy.

Most of the controversy is due to ignorance, the lack of research, and the fact, in most instances, the experts have never eaten real bread. It is their inability to differentiate between what constitutes real bread and evil bread, which is an impostor, masquerading as real bread, and by that, I mean everyday white, wholemeal, and multigrain bread.

The information in this book is rare, it includes some of the unpublished works of Professor Louis Kevran author of the book Bread's biological transmutation. It is also, a collation of the studies and works of other great scientists, bakers, and ancestors, who dedicated their lives to the quest for better bread.

This information needs to be passed on to future generations so they may know the truth behind, what constitutes real bread, what constitutes evil bread, and how they can flourish by being able to bake and eat real bread, a real nourishing food, which is why it was called "The staff of life". It was our first superfood.

You will be surprised at the ancient secrets of baking sourdough and allergy-free bread, that could well have been lost, forever, had this book not been written. You will be even more surprised to discover, very few people have ever eaten, real sourdough, allergy-free bread.

This bread book explains the simplicity of the laws of nature and how real honest-to-goodness bread baking fits perfectly into those laws of nature.

Being able to bake your own bread from start to finish is a valuable life skill that will give you the knowledge that will last a lifetime and ensure you and your family never go hungry. It will give you an unfair advantage over people who eat white or wholemeal bread and processed food.

Many people have a problem with eating imposter bread, like wheat or gluten intolerance allergies, poor digestion, intestinal problems, bloating, weight gain, high blood sugar levels, etc., but it is not real bread that causes those problems, rather, its everyday white, wholemeal and multigrain bread, the ingredients of which have been pillaged, plundered and laced with herbicides and chemicals, that cause the problems. These are not real bread, they are impostor bread masquerading as real bread, and continued eating of those bread will lead to allergic reactions and long-term health issues.

Our ancestors didn't have a problem eating bread, it was a staple food with every meal. Why do we? Maybe it's the fact that in his greed and quest for money, man has plundered, pillaged, and demineralized bread to the point it should not be called bread because it is an impostor masquerading as bread.

Fortunately, however, these people with allergies and intolerance to bread, no longer have to suffer from those problems once they know how to bake real sourdough, allergy-free bread. That's what you will learn about in this book. Specifically, you'll learn how to prepare and bake real, honest-to-goodness sourdough bread, from start to finish, the same bread that provided our ancestors with better nutrition and energy than any other food they ate.

Baking your own bread will provide you with the feeling of being a pioneer in the food industry, having discovered a secret food that few people know about, a food so nutritious and so simple and easy to prepare, you will be surprised, why the so-called experts haven't discovered it before.

Religious and sacred records embody valuable directions for the survival of the human race. Learning from these texts and practicing the directions given allows our intuition to acquire much-needed survival skills.

There is a sacred duty to point these truths out to our neighbors. Give a man a fish, feed him for a day, teach him how to fish, and feed him for a lifetime. That adage or Chinese proverb applies to bread. If we give a loaf of bread that we have baked to someone, we have only assured his or her sustenance for a day. By teaching that same person to bake their own, we have assured that person and his or her kinfolk a lifetime supply of the staff of life.

The advantages of milling your own grain and baking bread at home are the only way you can safely ensure that all the ingredients present in your real bread are pure, whole, and made without the use of processing aids or any other artificial additives.

Being able to bake your own bread from start to finish, including milling the grain to make the flour, mixing and kneading the dough, and ultimately baking the bread, will provide you with a great sense of satisfaction.

I grew up in an era (1950's and 1960's) when bread was a staple with every meal. Where wheat, gluten, and other intolerance and allergies were rare. Where people were healthy and rarely went to the doctor. I saw firsthand the impact a good loaf of bread had on the family's health and budget.

We dedicate this book to all people who have contributed in some way to making real bread the most nutritious and satiating food on the planet.

WHOLE GRAIN, SOURDOUGH WHEAT BREAD, WAS OUR FIRST SUPERFOOD IT STILL IS

CONTROVERSY OVER BREAD

There has been a lot of controversy about wheat bread over the last couple of decades or so, and it has been initiated mainly by the so-called experts and spin doctors. They malign real wheat bread, saying there is no difference between any bread, white or whole-grain bread and they all cause wheat or gluten intolerance allergies, poor digestion, intestinal problems, bloating, weight gain, high blood sugar levels, high glycemic index (GI) rating, and the list goes on, when in fact nothing could be further from the truth.

Most of the controversy is due to ignorance, the inability to differentiate between what makes up real bread and an impostor bread masquerading as real bread, and by that, I mean everyday white, wholemeal, and multigrain bread.

When I went to school 100% meant just that, whole, nothing deducted from or subtracted from that figure. Well, apparently that does not apply to bread. To many bakers and manufacturers, the word bread takes on the same meaning, that all bread is equal, and made the same way, there is nothing different between 100% organic whole grain sourdough bread (where nothing has been removed from the flour, nothing added) and yeasted white bread (where 30% the bran and germ and starch has been removed). Doesn't add up does it, doesn't sound right and you don't need a degree to work it out.

Now that's where the problem starts, the spin doctors and experts make their millions because they write books that discuss the harmful effects of white bread but use sleight of hand wording to make out that 100% organic whole grain sourdough bread has the same health issues as white bread, now that's deceitful.

WHY ALL THE COMMOTION

There is no problem, in terms of allergies or intolerance from eating real bread and we don't include people with diagnosed coeliac disease. It wasn't a problem for our ancestors in the past; it is not a problem for us now. In saying that I am talking about real bread that our ancestors ate, bread made from three ingredients, wheat, water, and salt, which was baked to a principle and a traditional baking process. I am not talking about everyday white, wholemeal, multigrain bread, we call them evil bread, impostors, masquerading as real bread and continued eating of that bread will lead to allergic reactions and long-term health issues. Follow the same bread-baking principle our ancestors used and say goodbye to allergies, and intolerance from eating bread.

That is why it is so important to bring people up to date with why impostor bread, not real bread causes many health issues and how they can take back their life and be able to eat real bread again with no reaction from allergies and intolerance, the bread our ancestors called the Staff of life, the same bread that successfully, built, advanced and sustained past civilizations. That is the exciting part.

Most of the so-called experts and spin doctors who malign real bread with no scientific validation to do so, have never eaten real whole grain wheat sourdough bread, and that applies to most people, so how can they pass judgment on something they have never tried and never allowed their body to respond to. That feeling is achieved by eating a super-food.

We need to give gratitude to our ancient civilizations, who chose wheat as their choice of grain. They all knew intuitively and had the common sense to realize that bread made from wheat sustained them better than any other food. They knew using sourdough as a leavening agent and the long fermentation process (a minimum of 8 hours) allowed the grain to pre-digest, so they had better assimilation and digestion on eating the bread made from it.

- They knew the long sourdough fermentation process, enabled all the nutrients from the grain to be extracted, unlike yeast that works so fast at leavening (rising) the dough, that there is not sufficient time to unlock the rich, life-giving minerals stored tightly within the bran coats. They knew going without their daily bread was the difference between living and starvation.

Organic wheat is the food richest in nutrition and energy, no other food, meat, milk, potatoes, fruits vegetables can equal the nutrition and energy that wheat supplies. So, on that basis, it is a no-brainer not to include organic whole wheat grain sourdough bread as a staple food in your diet. If humanity is to be strong, its staple food has to be wheat in bread form, we must free wheat from the commercial orientation that agri-business strives to monopolize and fight in order to preserve the older non-hybridized strains.

Wheaten bread was and still is our first superfood. 100% Whole wheat grain sourdough bread (real bread) contains more nutrients per weight than, meat, milk, potatoes, fruits, and vegetables" (Thomas, 1976). It is full of nutrition and energy, and it would supply a 25-49-year-old man with 30% of his energy requirements and 49% of his protein requirements" (Health & Welfare, 1990).

Man can almost live on real bread alone. Real bread organic whole grain wheat sourdough bread (not your everyday bread) contains the seven major dietary elements (calcium, phosphorous, potassium, sulfur, sodium, chlorine, magnesium) and most of the trace minerals all of which are so necessary to allow the human body to work efficiently and along with a few additional vegetables to sustain life.

Our ancestors didn't have the problems associated with their everyday bread, problems like wheat and gluten intolerance, allergies, bloating, weight gain, and high blood sugar levels because they used just three ingredients to make their bread, freshly milled wheaten flour, freshwater, and salt, nothing added, and nothing removed. They adhered to a traditional sourdough baking process based on the integrity of the ingredients which eliminated the allergy factors associated with eating everyday bread and allowed the dough to be thoroughly pre-digested through fermentation, so their own digestive system didn't have to work overtime to digest the whole grain bread.

GREED

The scientific evidence on real bread's nutritional benefits has been validated by our great European scientists, so why try to reinvent the wheel, why try to change a winning formula that has served civilization so well for thousands of years and the answer is GREED. You see making real bread is a commitment, the baking process takes time, a good loaf of sourdough bread will take anywhere from 8 to 18 hours from start to finish and today's bakers cannot afford that time or commitment, time is money to them. They want bread prepared and ready to bake within 30 minutes to an hour and will use whatever means it takes to do so, and that includes, pillaging, plundering, and demineralizing the flour, which includes bleaching, removal of the bran and germ, and the addition of chemicals, emulsifiers, and processing aids. This is not bread, it is a poor substitute, and the public are the guinea pigs that suffer as a result, and you don't have to.

Having made the comment about the baking process taking time, you can easily reduce your commitment time without interfering with the integrity of the baking process. This baking process will work for you, not you working for the process and I will discuss that further in the section on how to make real bread.

WHAT CONSTITUTES REAL BREAD

BY DEFINITION

The biggest problem surrounding the myth, that bread is bad for you, is the notion all bread is the same, made equal, and the ingredients and baking process are the same or with a minor difference. That could not be further from the truth and that is the problem, the misleading information that has led to confusion among people, about whether bread is good for you.

Real bread, that being 100% organic whole wheat grain sourdough bread is a complex carbohydrate and is highly beneficial for your health and wellbeing.

The Real Bread Campaign is a worldwide organization based in the United Kingdom and run by the charity Sustain. Its mission is to find and share ways to make bread better for us, better for our communities, and better for the planet. Their definition is "Real Bread" is made without the use of processing aids or any additives. It believes that any bread product with additives should not be called bread.

Let's put the record straight so there can be no more confusion. Real leavened bread, as made by our ancestors for thousands of years, was made with 3 ingredients:

1. 100% freshly milled organic whole grain wheat flour. (Today, the organic wheat kernel is kept by organic farmers and used each year for their seed. It has not been genetically modified, and no chemicals are used during the seeding, right through to the harvesting of the grain, either on the fields or on the grain. Our ancestors never used chemicals to grow their wheat.

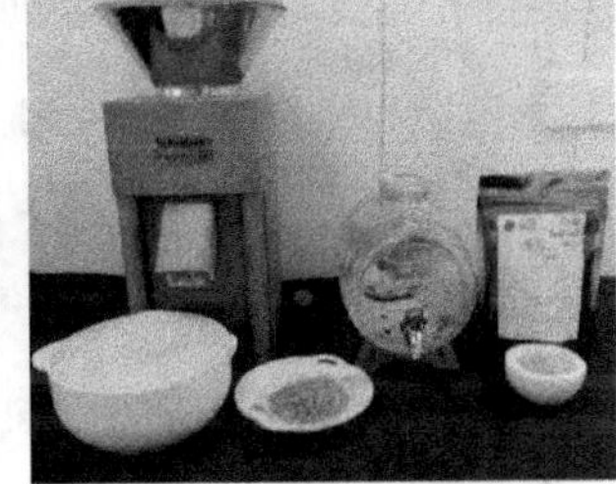

2. Filtered water.

3. Natural grey sea salt. (Celtic sea salt is the only salt to be scientifically validated to contain 84 minerals.)

The sourdough starter, the leavening agent that makes the bread rise before baking, is made from flour, water, and airborne microorganisms.

Nothing is removed from the flour (the bran, germ, and starch remain intact).

Nothing is added, by that I mean, dough conditioners, flour improvers, processing aids, chemical leavening, or any other artificial additives.

Sometimes, you might not want a plain loaf - you might want it enriched or otherwise jazzed up a bit.

Additional ingredients are great as long as they are natural (e.g., seeds, nuts, cheese, milk, malt extract, herbs, oils, fats, and dried fruits) and contain no artificial additives.

WHY NO ADDITIVES

Simply put, Real Bread doesn't need them. However, manufacturers may present their reasons in terms of consumer demand, their motivation for adulterating their products is generating greater profit.

Examples of the purposes of additives include:

- ❖ Prolonging the time, a loaf stays soft by artificial means and advertising this as 'freshness'.
- ❖ Spraying of chemical fungicides to prevent mold.
- ❖ Adapting natural ingredients to comply with the technical demands of modern processing.
- ❖ Modifying and supplementing natural ingredients to produce a certain type of product, rather than allowing the flour to determine the type of bread that can be produced.
- ❖ Shortening natural rising times

REAL BREAD'S MOST DEFINING CHARACTERISTIC

Real bread's most defining characteristic that sets it apart, is the fact it is fresh and tastes great, and will satiate you better than any other food, it takes away your hunger, nutritionally fills you up, and satisfies you from one meal to the next, with no allergic reaction. It satisfies your sweet cravings and takes away the need to snack in between meals.

The proof is always in the eating, and this is one way to prove beyond doubt the point that our ancestors have made, that real bread provides complete appetite satisfaction when you eat it. These qualities separate real bread, from your everyday impostor bread, which will fill you up for an hour, maybe two, then you're hungry again.

Once you eat bread, made from freshly milled flour, you will never go back to eating everyday bread, made with stale, rancid, dead flour, that is well past its use-by date. Freshly milled 100% whole grain wheat flour, tastes sweet, and that sweet taste is replicated in the baked loaf. You will experience a feeling of total satisfaction, a feeling of your body responding to the food of outstanding quality, that will provide nutrition and energy to last you from one meal to the next without the need to snack. It is as if you are a pioneer; you have discovered a secret food that no one else knows about, food that gives you an unfair advantage over people eating every day, white and wholemeal bread, a food so simple and effective, you wonder why the so-called experts haven't discovered it before you.

WHAT REAL BREAD IS NOT

Bread is the oldest and most widely manufactured food. Because it has been around for such a long time, many ways to exploit it for profit have been invented and many detrimental practices have crept into its production, more than any other food.

All commercial flour today is produced by large milling corporations. Processed "patent" flour is customarily stripped of the essential substances in the germ, the bran, and its oil. This wanton degeneration and emasculation of the flour endanger the health of the consumer.

The giant milling industry uses high-tech industrial mills. This process also loads the finished white patent product with dangerous chemical additives. Both the mechanical and the chemical procedures out-vie each other to sterilize the flour so that it can be shipped, untouched by bugs and free of any natural biological breakdown, across continents and still pretend to have a long shelf life.

It is important to review the negative effects of additives. Many things are added to white patent flour, but even more, chemicals are added to supermarket whole wheat flour. This is because these dark flours are more appetizing than white flour to worms and weevils and require a larger dose of chemicals to ward off infestations from these insects. Also, wholemeal flour requires more preservatives since it still contains nutrients and oils that could cause rancidity with aging.

Everyday bread (white, wholemeal, and multigrain bread) is made with commercial flour. It is a refined carbohydrate and is made using, yeast and artificial additives, it is not real bread and is not beneficial to your health and can lead to serious health issues and obesity.

So, if the bread you are eating is everyday white, wholemeal, or multigrain bread, made with commercial flour, where the bran and germ are removed from the flour, and the following ingredients are added to the bread mix, dough conditioners, flour improvers, processing aids, chemical leavening, or any other artificial additives, it ain't real bread.

If bread gives you allergic reactions, bloat, indigestion, constipation, high sugar levels, and if you gain weight by eating it, it ain't real bread, it's that simple.

THE FIRST LOST ANCIENT SECRET

WHY ORGANIC WHEAT GRAIN MUST BE USED TO MAKE OUR BREAD

How could anyone ignore the fact, that, if some 80-odd chemicals and additives are added to the process of manufacturing bread, it won't have a huge bearing on allergies and intolerance from eating everyday, white, whole meal, and multigrain bread.

What most of the so-called bread experts forgot to mention in their bread analysis is that wheat or gluten is not the problem, rather it's the herbicides and chemicals that are sprayed on the crops that make the bread, that are the problem. There can be as many as 80 chemicals added to a loaf of bread, from the milling of the grain to the finished loaf of bread. Don't you think that might have an impact on allergies and intolerance to eating a loaf of that bread?

According to Dr. Zach Bush, one of the few triples board-certified physicians in the USA, and a specialist in the gut (microbiome) and glyphosate research, and founder of farmers footprint a non for profit organization teaching regenerative farming techniques. He believes, herbicides could end life on Earth. Roundup (glyphosate) is probably our public enemy number one, but that's one of 260 chemicals that are now prevalent in our food system. It is possible that we're beyond the recovery of the human species, where we've got maybe 60 or 70 years left as a species at our current trajectory of collapse, because of chemicals like glyphosate? More than that, because of everything we're doing.

We are currently spraying 5.5 billion pounds of toxic glyphosate a year (approx. 2.5 billion tonnes) around the planet and at that rate, it must impact our lives. life at that rate is not sustainable for the long-term survival of the human race.

In addition to that, there are now many genetically modified wheat crops in existence. They've been genetically modified to be able to be sprayed directly with this chemical glyphosate.

There was only a small number of people suffering from wheat allergies, celiac disease, and gluten sensitivity before 1992, that's when they started spraying roundup (glyphosate) on wheat crops. Within a couple of years of that, we had an epidemic of wheat allergies called, celiac disease and gluten sensitivity. We invented gluten- sensitivity, out of the application of glyphosate, or roundup to this gluten-containing wheat.

Since that time, wheat and gluten sensitivity has escalated dramatically and of course, the experts blame wheat, or gluten for the problem, which is totally incorrect. You are not gluten intolerant, you are roundup (glyphosate) intolerant.

Roundup (glyphosate) is one culprit, if not the biggest problem, it acts as an antibiotic to kill the microbial diversity in your intestines. It causes a lack of oxygen in the gut lining, and that hypoxic injury up-regulates the receptor for gliadin, which is the breakdown product of gluten, which then causes permeability (leaking) of the gut lining.

This epidemic of chronic disease has emerged from this collapse of the microbiome. Your gut membrane is the largest barrier to the outside world, it covers two tennis courts in surface area and is the thickness of half of the width of a human hair. So, it's this tiny, microscopic cellophane-like covering that separates the outside world from your human biology.

What glyphosate and Roundup does is perforate that membrane by destroying those tight junctions, (tight junctions are the junctions or the seal or joint between two cells in the epithelial membrane. In simple words, they prevent leakage), and creating something – that's now called "leaky gut". In the medical literature it's called gut permeability, it increases gut permeability.

That injury activates the immune system, and we become reactive to our foods. So, we develop allergies of all sorts, pollen allergies, and environmental allergies, but also all the food allergies, such as wheat and gluten intolerance, that have become so prevalent in our children today. And so, we lose the front-line defense barrier in our immune system, which allows all forms of chemicals, herbicides, bacteria, and viruses, to enter our bodies with no resistance. So, at that point, not only have you become chronically inflamed, but you're also literally losing self-identity.

We now spray many of our staple crops, the legumes, the lentils, and the beans with glyphosate. So many other things are being sprayed now with glyphosate, just like wheat, not to kill weeds, but to dry the crop quicker. We use them as a desiccant. That desiccating process means that we're spraying the crop hours or days before harvest, which means that the individual is going to get very high residues of those chemicals.

Glyphosate is the active ingredient in the popular weed killer Roundup and about 500 other herbicide products. In some studies Roundup, the world's most widely used herbicide has also been linked to other health problems, these include, Hodgkin lymphoma, Liver damage, Diabetes, Kidney disease, Parkinson's disease, Breathing problems, Lou Gehrig's disease, Sterility in men.

So if you are eating non-organic, everyday, white, wholemeal, or multigrain bread, biscuits. cakes, breakfast cereals, and pasta, there is a great chance you are eating GMO bread to start with, which has been sprayed with roundup (glyphosate). Maybe now you can reason why you are intolerant and allergic to bread and other non-organic food products and are experiencing health problems such as wheat or gluten intolerance, allergies, poor digestion, intestinal problems, IBS, leaky gut, bloating, saliva burns in the mouth and throat, nausea, vomiting, and diarrhea.

Organic farming is a method of crop and livestock production that involves much more than choosing not to use pesticides, fertilizers, genetically modified organisms, antibiotics, and growth hormones.

Organic production is a holistic system designed to optimize the productivity and fitness of diverse communities within the Agroecosystem, including soil organisms, plants, livestock, and people. The principal goal of organic production is to develop enterprises that are sustainable and harmonious with the environment.

Organic farming was the method used by our ancestors to grow wheat and other grains. They never called it organic, it was called natural farming and was based on the same principle as organic, as they never sprayed chemicals on their crops, never removed the bran and germ from the flour that made their bread, and never used artificial additives when making bread. The result of organic or natural farming used by our ancestors was, they rarely had allergies and intolerance from eating real bread and their health was so much better than people today, who eat everyday white, wholemeal and multigrain bread.

That's why it is imperative, we eat bread and associated products, like biscuits, cakes, slices, and pasta, made with organic whole grain flour (free from herbicides and chemicals), or organic wheat, which is milled and made into bread and associated products, to avoid long-term health problems, and the recovery and sustainability of our land and planet.

THE SECOND LOST ANCIENT SECRET

THE NUTRITIONAL IMPORTANCE OF BRAN & GERM IN BREAD

If you want to stop allergies and intolerance that come about from eating bread, only eat whole grain bread, that has not had the bran and germ removed from it, is made without chemicals, and without the use of processing aids or any other artificial additives. It's that simple.

The kernel of wheat is composed of the outer bran layer, the germ, and the endosperm. It is rich in nutrients, which include vitamins A, B, C, D, and E, which are concentrated in the bran and germ. Of special importance is that it contains the entire B complex, except for vitamin B12. B vitamins function as cofactors in many metabolic reactions involved in the release of energy (Birdsall, 1985).

The bran and germ are the most important, and most nutritional part of flour that makes bread. When you remove them or part of them from the flour, that makes bread, which is the case with everyday white, wholemeal, and multi-grain bread, you take away the driving force, the most nutritional parts of bread, that help sustain you from one meal to the next. That has a huge impact on your health.

When all the ingredients in whole grain organic flour are kept in a whole state, nothing is removed and the bran and germ remain in their natural, original proportions and, nothing is added, which means the bread is made without chemicals, and without the use of processing aids or any other artificial additives, good things happen.

It allows the seven major dietary elements, calcium, phosphorous, potassium, sulfur, sodium, chlorine, magnesium, and the trace elements present in whole grain flour to do the job nature intended them to do, that being to provide the human body with optimum nutrition so it can sustain itself from being hungry for long periods and without any allergic reactions.

The germ, which includes the scutellum, is especially rich in vitamins, B, and E, high-quality protein, unsaturated fats, minerals, and carbohydrates.

Niacin is a B3 vitamin, it is such an important vitamin, it is essential for good health, and is present naturally in whole grain bread. It has been proven to be very effective against mental illness, stress, anxiety, sleeplessness, nutritional deficiency, joint pain, and arthritic issues, and they remove bad cholesterol from the body.

A study at the University of California, at Irvine (Gutierrez), and over forty years of research by Dr. Abram Hoffer showed, that niacin, a B3 vitamin, lowers, low-density lipoprotein (bad cholesterol), elevates high-density lipoprotein HDL (good cholesterol), and reduces the ravages of heart disease.

In 2007, the New York Times, reported, that inexpensive vitamin B3, niacin, can increase HDL (good cholesterol) as much as 35 percent, when taken in doses usually about 2000 milligrams per day (4 x 500mg capsules). It also lowers and removes LDL (bad cholesterol) and triglycerides by as much as 50 percent. Niacin vitamin B3 absorbs cholesterol in the blood and carries it back to the liver. The liver then flushes it from the body.

The New York Times quoted, Steven E. Nissen M.D., president of the American College of Cardiology, as saying, "Niacin, is really it. Nothing else available is that effective" for removing cholesterol from the body.

Niacin was first used to successfully lower serum cholesterol in 1955. Since then, placebo-controlled studies have confirmed that niacin vitamin B3, prevents second heart attacks, and niacin also reduces strokes. One study showed, that after fifteen years, men taking niacin, had an 11 percent lower death rate.

Diets high in complex carbohydrates such as whole-wheat bread and cereal grains, legumes, and vegetables are usually the custom in populations with a very low incidence of cardiovascular disease (Brown et al, 1985). Studies indicate that high-fiber diets decrease blood pressure in normal as well as hypertensive subjects (Birdsall,1985). For elevated blood serum lipids dietary recommendations include increasing carbohydrate consumption to make up 65% of total daily calories, emphasizing complex carbohydrates from nature, sources (Gotto et al., 1984).

The bran is rich in fiber, minerals, vitamin B6, thiamine, folate, vitamin E, and some phytochemicals, in particular, antioxidants such as phenolic compounds (Shewry, 2009).

Other vitamins and numerous other minerals are found in the bran and germ part of a wheat kernel, though in small amounts. These include carotene, vitamin B6 or pyridoxine, pantothenic acid, biotin, and folic acid, vitamin C, and vitamin K. Other minerals are sodium, calcium, chlorine, manganese, zinc, copper, cobalt, nickel, chromium, molybdenum, fluoride, iodine, boron, selenium, lead, aluminum, and silicon oxide (Souci, 1981). The body is capable of converting the carotene to produce one-sixth its amount as vitamin A (Health ~ Welfare, 1990).

Can you see now why our ancestors were so much healthier than we are today and had less allergies and intolerance to bread. The bread they ate was whole grain, with nothing taken from it and nothing added to it. Their diet was high carb, high-fat diet and bread was a staple with every meal. They ate chemical-free fruit and vegetables, usually grown in their own gardens. Heart disease, cancer, obesity, and diabetes were not major health issues like they are today, and people rarely went to the doctor and antibiotics were only given in emergencies. Can we not learn from history? You cannot pillage, plunder, and demineralize flour, to make bread and expect a positive outcome.

THE ALLERGY PROBLEM

When the bran and germ have been removed from the flour, which is the case with everyday white, wholemeal, and multigrain bread, it results in an average loss of 70-80% of nutrients that are present in the bran and germ, and should not be equated with wholesomeness (Davis, 1981) The consumption of everyday, white, wholemeal, or multigrain bread, clearly places the body at a disadvantage, casting a burden on the rest of the diet (Pomeranz, 1988).

Many allergic reactions and intolerances caused by eating everyday bread are the results of what man does to the flour that makes the bread, not wheat or gluten. There is a substance, an ester in all grains, particularly wheat called phytic acid. People do not realize how much of a problem phytic acid is, it is rarely discussed, and yet it poses real health issues that no one is addressing.

Phytic acid cannot be removed from everyday yeasted bread (white, wholemeal, multigrain bread), because yeast is not a true ferment, and commercial bakers use flour that has had the bran and germ removed from it. In so doing, they have removed the enzyme called phytase, which nature has provided in the bran part of wheat grain, to neutralize, and eliminate the phytic acid.

Phytic acid, is known as a food inhibitor, it can be toxic in large doses, it is present in the starchy part of white bread at a rate of 90 milligrams per 100 grams of bread and in wholemeal and multigrain bread in varying degrees. As long as the bran which houses the enzyme called phytase has not been removed from the bread, phytic acid will be naturally, neutralized, and there is no risk of poisoning or mineral deficiency.

When the bran has been removed from bread which is the case with everyday bread, phytic acid blocks the absorption of many crucial minerals into our body, minerals like phosphorus, zinc, iron, calcium, magnesium, and manganese, and can lead to mineral deficiencies. It can slow down the metabolism, which is so crucial to weight loss in burning calories and can result in rickets (vitamin C deficiency) and osteoporosis occurring. Phytic acid is responsible for many of the allergies, and intolerance associated with eating everyday bread.

In addition, commercial bakers of everyday bread, do not allow their breads to proof (allow the dough to, rest, and mature before baking) for a period of 8 hours which is the minimum period to eliminate the phytic acid from the bread.

People who consume foods high in phytic acids, such as grain, seeds, nuts, beans, some fruits, and vegetables such as berries, green beans, and potatoes as a major source of calories and do not follow the proper ancestral procedure of activating these foods to neutralize and eliminate the phytic acid content from them, can be subject to real health problems, such as vitamin and mineral deficiencies, allergic reactions, high blood sugar levels, slow metabolism, weight gain, bloat, poor digestion, constipation, gluten intolerance to name a few.

Activating flour to neutralize the phytic acid effect in bread, means not removing the bran and germ from flour and allowing the bread mix to rest for at least 8 hours, before placing it in the oven to bake. Activating, for seeds, nuts, beans, some fruits, and vegetables such as berries, green beans, and potatoes, means, soaking overnight, or for 8 hours.

Can you see now why our ancestors were so much healthier than we are today and had less allergies and intolerance to bread. They followed the rule of nature, not man. The bread they ate was whole grain. All the ingredients, including the bran and germ, were kept in a whole state, nothing was removed, and nothing added like chemicals, processing aids, or any other artificial additives.

Their diet was high carb, high-fat diet and bread was a staple with every meal. They ate chemical-free fruit and vegetables, usually grown in their own gardens. Heart disease, cancer, obesity, and diabetes were not major health issues like they are today, and people rarely went to the doctor and antibiotics were only given in emergencies. Can we not learn from history? You cannot pillage, plunder, and demineralize flour, to make bread and expect a positive outcome.

THE THIRD LOST ANCIENT SECRET

RANCID, STALE, DEAD BREAD, YOU'RE EATING IT

It may seem incredible to believe, but it's true, very few people have ever tasted a loaf of real sourdough bread made from 100% organic whole wheat grain flour, freshly milled on the baker's premises and used immediately to make bread, nothing removed from the mix, especially the bran & germ and nothing added to it, and by that I mean, made without the use of processing aids or any other artificial additives.

Your everyday, white, wholemeal or multigrain bread, and even organic sourdough bread, is not made with freshly milled flour, it is made with stale, rancid, dead flour, well past its use-by date (that is flour that has been milled 1- 6 months, even longer before use) and that difference alone is massive in the overall bread-making process.

Some people are pedantic about checking use-by dates on food labels in supermarkets, yet overlook the fact, that the flour used to make everyday bread and associated products, like, cakes, biscuits, pasta, are well past their use-by dates. The flour used to make these products is stale, dead, and rancid approximately 95% of the time. You wouldn't eat a rotten apple, but people are eating stale, rancid, dead, bread, cakes, biscuits, and pasta, and don't even realize it, or don't care to do something about it.

As an analogy, consider an apple. Cut up and crush an apple, once its skin is broken, the inside soon blackens and decays. The same happens to any whole grain kernel, once it has been milled, cracked, or rolled, even though it doesn't visibly blacken after milling, it does however immediately begin to decay and loses more of its nutrients the longer it is exposed to the elements. Freshly milled grain is stale 3 days after grinding. You wouldn't eat a rotten apple, yet you eat stale and rancid, dead bread because most people don't know any better. Over 95% of all bread, cakes, biscuits, pasta, etc. are made with stale, rancid, dead flour. No wonder bread has lost its popularity because it has been demineralized and laced with chemicals.

ADVANTAGES OF FRESH FLOUR

Anyone who has smelled organic whole grain flour, freshly ground, will be well aware of its superior fragrance. The taste is sweet and delicious, and once you taste it, you will never go back to eating bread made with stale, dead, rancid flour or using packaged flour, which is stale and dead by comparison, for any of your baking requirements.

The nutritional importance of using fresh stone-ground grains for bread-making was revealed in the results of feeding studies in Germany (Bernasek, 1970). Rats that were fed diets comprising 50% flour or bread. Group 1 consumed freshly milled stone-ground flour. They fed group 2 bread made with this flour. Group 3 consumed the same flour as Group 1 but after 15 days of storage. Group 4 was fed bread made from flour fed to Group 3. A fifth group consumed white flour.

After four generations, only the rats fed freshly milled, fresh stone-ground flour, and those fed the bread made with it maintained their fertility. The rats in groups 3 to 5 had become infertile. Four generations for rats are believed to be equivalent to one hundred years in humans.

Your everyday, white, wholemeal & multi-grain bread, made from flour that is stale, rancid, dead, past its use-by date, that has been in storage for long periods, could well be another reason it is becoming more difficult for women to conceive.

Different ecological standards for flour storage set limits of 15 to 60 days (Picker & Pederson, 1990), although rancidity has been detected as early as 2 to 14 days after milling (Larsen, 1988). Freshly milled flour is old, and rancid, three days after grinding (Kervran, 1970).

HOW COMMERCIAL FLOUR FOR EVERYDAY BREAD IS PRODUCED

Bread is the oldest and most widely manufactured food. Because it has been around for such a long time, many ways to exploit it for profit have been invented and numerous detrimental practices have crept into its production, more than any other food.

Most of the commercial flour today is produced by large milling corporations. Processed "patent" flour is customarily stripped of the essential substances contained in the germ, the bran, and its oil. This wanton degeneration and emasculation of the flour endangers the health of the consumer.

The giant milling industry uses high-tech industrial mills. This process also loads the finished white patent product with dangerous chemical additives. Both the mechanical and the chemical procedures outvie each other to sterilize the flour so that it can be shipped, untouched by bugs and free of any natural biological breakdown, across continents and still pretend to have a long shelf life.

It is important to review the negative effects of additives. many things are added to white patent flour, but even more, chemicals are added to supermarket whole wheat flour. This is because these dark flours are more appetizing than white flour to worms and weevils and require a larger dose of chemicals to ward off infestations from these insects. Also, whole wheat flour requires more preservatives since it still contains nutrients and oils that could cause rancidity with aging.

One should be very wary of these additives, most of them have never been adequately tested for potential toxicity, yet the consumer is lulled into feeling safe because they are labelled GRAS, or " generally recognised as safe." They are used liberally in today's commercial bread. As many as 80 different chemicals can be incorporated into a single fancy loaf and the law does not require that these be individually mentioned on the bread wrappers list of ingredients.

Preservatives are a good case in point, even a yeasted loaf of commercial bread retains a life of its own and will go on living inside the plastic casket or wrapper. A way to stop the growth of bacteria, fungus, and spores by using chemicals was devised and serves to still the microbial life before it causes cosmetic problems such as green or orange molds forming in bread, crust and crumb. These also effectively and permanently prevent human digestion of the same loaf.

Some of the toxic chemicals include mercurial, methyl bromide, chlorine dioxide gas and nitrogen trichloride, these last two are used to bleach "age", condition and preserve the sterility of the flour. Whiteners include alum, chalk ammonium carbonate and nitrogen peroxide.

"Aged flour" is a euphemistic term employed by the milling trade to describe their old "fossilized" and depleted flour. propaganda aimed at bakers infers that, for them, aged flour works best. Aging is a catalyst for oxidation, however, and it destroys all vitamins and enzymes.

When these elements are gone, only the calories remain. In order to compensate for this flagrant deficiency, the US government has made the enriching process mandatory. To "protect" and "help" the consumer, synthetic vitamins, such as Thiamine, riboflavin and niacin, must be added along with iron.

Considering how little is known about the absorption of iron and niacin fortification well above the level nature intended, constitutes an unproven nutritional experiment of unprecedented scale.

Most bakers and all bread and pasta factories around the world add even more chemicals during the mixing of the dough. Some of these additives attempt to overcome the obvious deadliness of flour. Dyes, anti-digest ants (preservatives), and plastic softeners help retard drying and staling. All of these are part of the arsenal of today's bakeries.

How can food-conscious consumers counter this runaway degeneration of an important staple food? The ideal solution is to re-learn home milling and baking and follow dietary guidelines set by tradition in all the wise past civilizations. Only then are we guaranteed that no emasculation of the flour has occurred, as well as a total absence of the fast buck expedient methods that have begun to destroy the fiber of mankind.

Whole wheat bread can once again be the richest, most economical source of human energy, provided it is made with care while using the traditional natural leaven method. Bread baking must be returned to the home fire where it has always belonged. The process of making pre-biblical bread with only three ingredients, wheat, water, and salt is considerably simpler than the delicate timing of yeasted bread. It is also the only nourishing, abundantly satisfying, and waste-free baking process worth practicing.

THE DIFFERENCE BETWEEN, WHOLE GRAIN, WHOLEMEAL AND WHITE BREAD

I would like to explain how the extraction of the bran and germ from the flour creates the three types of bread, whole grain, wholemeal and white bread and how that factor alone creates a vast difference between 100% whole grain sourdough bread and what we know as everyday bread (White, Wholemeal multigrain bread).

When you hear the term 100% extraction rate flour, it means the flour is 100% pure, with nothing removed from it and it has retained all the bran, germ, and tougher outer layers of endosperm in it. Higher extraction flour is darker than wholemeal or white flour. So, the term 100% extraction refers to 100% whole grain flour that makes whole grain bread.

When the bran and germ are removed from the wheat berry on milling, you have flour which is 85% extraction, as the bran makes up approximately 12% of the mass of the wheat berry and the germ roughly 3%. The term 85% extraction usually refers to your everyday wholemeal or multigrain bread.

The flour that is 85% extraction, is fairly coarse and dark and needs further sifting of the coarse parts of the flour to get it to what is known as 70% extraction flour, or what we refer to as everyday white bread.

Even today in some parts of Europe they still use the old system of determining the amount of extraction in flour by burning the flour to determine the amount of extraction. 55 centigrams of ashes per 100 grams of flour will be equivalent to 74% extraction (white flour) and 110 centigrams of ashes per 100 grams of flour correspond to an 85% extraction (wholemeal or multigrain flour).

COMPARISON OF CONTENTS BETWEEN: WHOLE GRAIN, SEMI-WHITE (WHOLEMEAL) & WHITE FLOUR

	True whole-grain flour 100-98% extraction	Semi white flour 80-85% extraction	White flour 70-75% extraction
Proteins	10%	10%	9.5%
Fats	1.5%	1.5%	1.2%
Carbohydrates	71%	72%	75%
Vitamins (in milligrams / 100grams of flour)			
B10	35mg	0.25mg	0.10mg
B2	0.20	0.15	0.08
C	25	0.20	00
Minerals			
Sulphur	180mg	100mg	60mg
Phosphorous	300	200	120
Chlorine	50	30	20
Sodium	10	6	3
Potassium	450	300	90
Magnesium	140	60	20
Magnesium in Rye	130	55	30
Calcium	40	24	16
Iron	4	2.5	1.2
Zinc	5.5	3.2	1.7
Copper	0.7	0.4	0.2
Manganese	3	1.8	0.9

(Breads biological transmutations by Professor Louis Kervran).

While the difference in the first 3 elements remains slight, the major minerals in the second part of the table show a rapid decrease when the extraction percent falls below 98%.

We now see why so-called whole meal, multigrain white, bread, cereals, pancake mixes, pasta, biscuits, and cakes are highly deficient and create many diseases in humans.

WHITE BREAD LEADS TO OBESITY

You can understand now the large nutritional difference that separates white bread from whole grain bread. White bread first leads to obesity, since its carbohydrates change into fats within the body. This stems from the fact that white flour contains 7 times less magnesium than whole grain flour. 100% whole grain wheat, sourdough bread builds muscle, not fat, and it does not cause weight gain. Nature has compounded a sufficient quantity of magnesium to maintain biological harmony. We have recognized a lack of magnesium as causing carbohydrates to change into fats, which translates into weight gain. So if you are eating everyday white, wholemeal, or multigrain bread, expect weight gain to happen, along with a host of health issues such as wheat or gluten intolerance, or allergies, poor digestion, intestinal problems, bloating, constipation, high blood sugar levels, and the list goes on.

Besides the mineral deficiencies, there is in white bread and almost wholesale lack of vitamins. Because of the total lack of Vitamin C in the white bread, the law compels the bakers to add it in the form of ascorbic acid. Ascorbic acid is not Vitamin C, despite what most of us have been led to believe. Ascorbic acid alone depletes vitamin C from the body and can be quite dangerous when given to people who are severely Vitamin C deficient.

Within the whole grain flour, there exists a complex of natural vitamin C called "pro-vitamin C" which is so stable that it resists temperatures 200 degrees Celsius (392 degrees Fahrenheit) so that even after baking, it remains alive and unchanged in the soft part of the loaf. Ordinary vitamin C (ascorbic acid) however is rapidly destroyed by the heat of 100 degrees Celsius (212 degrees Fahrenheit), therefore it disappears from cooked vegetables and meat.

The pro-vitamin C is found in the second outside coat of the grain, the nonporous Epicarp. There also are found the B1, B2, and the PP vitamins (Niacin B3 in the form of nicotinic acid). However, both the D and E vitamins are within the germ. Note also that the fermentation of the dough in sourdough bread creates an important increase in the B complex vitamins.

Whilst it would appear you could almost live on real bread alone and the fact that it is a superfood in its own right, a diet based on grain alone would be unbalanced and unsustainable, it requires an additional complement of vegetables.

Are you starting to see already, that when we stray from our ancestral heritage of baking to a tried-and-true bread-baking principle, health issues develop? White bread has very little nutritional value, it is starch. What many people still ignore is the fact that white bread causes many diseases of civilization since bread is still the base of our food supply, now ruled by chemistry rather than biological considerations.

COMPARING VITAMIN PERCENTAGES IN WHOLE GRAIN WHEAT BREAD AGAINST WHITE BREAD

Extraction percent	Whole Grain Bread 98-100%	White Bread 70-75%
Vitamin E (Tocopherol)	1.30 mg	0.20 mg
Vitamin PP (Niacin B3 in the form of Nicotinio acid)	3.0	0.5

Most of the vitamin PP in white bread comes from that in the chemically active yeast.

YEAST IN ANCIENT HISTORY

When Moses told his people to commemorate the Exodus by partaking in unleavened (yeast-free) bread, it was not the first time that the Jewish people were advised to bake without yeast. The custom of eating unyeasted bread is much older than Moses and based on considerations of more significance than the mere commemoration of a historical event.

Much earlier when Lot received the angels of the Lord (Genesis 19:3) "and he did bake unleavened bread, and they ate", the dietary law requiring the consumption of unyeasted bread was already firmly established.

There is much evidence that humanity has repeatedly shunned yeasted bread. In Rome's pre-Christian religion, the flamen dialis, the priest of Jupiter, was forbidden to touch "*Fariam fermento imbutam*" a flour product containing yeast, thus setting a precedent for our recently acquired knowledge of the health dangers of yeast.

The Celtic people, prior to their conquest by the Roman hordes, obeyed the ritual of their ancient tradition and offered wheat, barley, and oat seeds to the poor at the time of the winter solstice. Then with the waxing season having begun, the Celtic celebration of the germination of the wheat took place.

"Eghi an ed" is still celebrated in French Canada as "Guignolee" and is still known in South American countries as "El Aguinaldo".

The Roman conquest scattered the Celts to the far corners of the earth, in Galicia (northwestern Spain) which received its share of the Celtic exodus, the chrysalis just freed from its cocoon is still named "aguinaldo" and it is this concept of the renewing of life that is celebrated by the descendants of the Celtic people everywhere at winter solstice's time.

The Druid priestesses paid great homage to the sublime secret of life and knew of the great similarities that existed between the human fetus in the first month of its life and the germinating grain of wheat. Their bread, both the daily and the sacramental, was leavened solely by the earth's forces.

King Louis XIV called a special council on the 24th of March 1668, to consider the objections to yeast that were being raised by his people. Seventy-five professors of the faculty of science were asked for their advice. After a lengthy discussion, thirty were for and forty-five were against using yeast at all. On August 13th, 1668, six doctors and six nobles were asked to give their ruling. The doctors were divided in their opinions, four were against yeast and two were for it. The nobles reserved their judgment but finally agreed.

Finally, after more discussion two years later, on March 21, 1670, Parliament permitted only the occasional use of brewer's yeast but strictly limited its use. They decreed that yeast from breweries could be used in Paris, but only if supplied by a brewer in that city, or from the immediate surrounding countryside. They further stipulated that the yeast be fresh and not adulterated in any way by additives and restricted its use to emergency situations. So you can see today, just like in the past, nothing has changed, anything passed by parliament can be stretched to the limit without any retribution if it serves self-interest and greed.

In Brittany today the dark wheat and buckwheat bread are still naturally leavened and pungent with the fragrance of the dark earth on the longest night of the year. In the heart of this region, in Vitre, the "Pain d'Antan" is still baked according to the Celto-Ligurian tradition of allowing the germ and its enzymes to leaven the bread to the exclusion of all yeast and any other leavening additives. And that is what we call REAL BREAD.

Celto-Ligure and its derivations: Lingons, Langre means "Fecund Earth" (productive) in Celtic

THE FOURTH LOST ANCIENT SECRET

WHY YEAST MUST BE TOTALLY AVOIDED IN BREAD

Modern times have launched the controversy of yeast versus natural leaven (sourdough), now natural leaven is winning and is backed up by scientific research.

During the first half of the twentieth century, most bakery experts maintained that neither leaven (sourdough) nor yeast had any advantage over the other and claimed that the two were interchangeable. False ideas such as these die slowly, even in the face of overwhelming evidence from the points of view of health, microbiology, and medicine.

To set the record straight, we will detail some biological and bio-electronic reasons yeast must be totally avoided in bread if it is to promote and maintain health.

Yeasted bread with its reduction, followed by oxidation, is totally opposed to the normal laws of life. At the natural culmination of this biological decay, the staling of the bread, deficient oxidative energy changes into a glycolized energy, as evidenced by "monster" or anarchistic type cells which exactly duplicate human cells experiencing grave illness. (This theory was presented by Otto Warburg, West Germany 1883-1970, discoverer of the yellow aerobic ferment, Nobel prize winner in 1931 for the study of fermentation and linkage to cancer).

Consuming yeasted whole wheat bread can encourage rickets (vitamin C deficiency), anemia, and bone decalcification. The danger of decalcification is totally eliminated, and chronic calcium deficiency is even corrected when the same whole wheat dough is naturally leavened.

(1) Yeast works so fast at leavening (rising) the dough that there is not sufficient time to unlock the rich, life-giving minerals stored tightly within the bran coats.

When the dough may leaven by itself, or by introducing a natural sourdough starter, which it will readily do if the flour is whole, of good biological quality, freshly ground, and unchemicalised, moisture absorption takes place to maximum capacity, allowing all the minerals to become freely available to human organism. This slower mode of panification, or dough maturing, enables an almost total pre-digestion of carbohydrates by enzyme development that cannot be achieved in yeasted bread. This helps digestion and prevents wheat allergies.

(2) When flour of any quality, whether treated, or untreated is mixed with yeast, it will combine to form phytic acid, a substance that prevents its fixation, or retainment by the body's metabolism of the essential elements offered initially by the whole wheat. It blocks mineral absorption, so the minerals are going straight down the toilet, rather than to the areas of the body where they are most needed.

In bread made with sourdough, the self-leavening process rises much more slowly than one produced with yeast. Its medium is favorable to the development of a beneficial phytase ferment, similar to the enzymes found in saliva. This phytase successfully neutralizes and eliminates the troublesome phytic acid so that all minerals liberated by the action mentioned in (1) are readily available to the organism.

(3) Professor Claude Louis Vincent founded The Bio-Electronic Research Center, located at, Avrille, France in 1961 and along with Dr J Rousseau researched biological and organic farming. They plotted the characteristics of unleavened versus the yeasted kind in terms of (pH) and oxido-reduction potential (rH). They have concluded that yeasted bread stales (less than 24 hours after baking), the rH factor rises from 25 to 32 millivolts. This is the toxic zone, they cite, cancer, polio, thrombosis, and arteriosclerosis as examples of conditions falling into this range.

Non-Yeasted bread increases in its alkalinity, the pH ranges from 6.5 to about 8 and the rH ranges from 18 to 25 microvolts. Improvement in flavor and taste occurs with each day and many people find that they prefer "older" bread, for at this point it becomes a true healing bread.

The "dry bread and water" method of healing the sick and those who broke the law, whether divine or man-made, was not intended as deprivation or punishment, it was therapy. Vigorous chewing of hard bread demands hard work from the masseter and temporal muscles, which stimulate the "good judgment" area of the brain, allowing the patient to regain his equilibrium and judgment and the prisoner to see his erring ways in a clear light.

The older non-yeasted sourdough bread gets better, the more its flavor and rejuvenating powers are increased. This is due to the lower oxido-reduction or rH factor. Because water content in non-yeasted sourdough bread remains stable, its bioelectrical resistivity remains constant.

(4) Yeast evolution within the dough medium destroys the nutritional elements in its environment. This loss of energy due to the yeast's consuming the starches is called glycolysis (the breaking down of carbohydrates) and benefits the all-consuming single-celled yeast organism saccharomyces.

Yeast is composed of just a single mushroom-like micro-organism, saccharomyces endomycetales, which consumes extraordinarily large amounts of energy and propagates itself in explosive bursts   Although the quantity of yeast added at the onset may be minimal, as in the yeast-based starters favored by health-minded bakers, as little as 50,000 yeast cells per gram will develop to the maximum count of 150,00,000 cells in each gram of mature, yeast saturated dough.

The growth curve of yeast duplicates that of the proliferation of cancer cells. To fuel this explosive reaction, the complex sugars (polysaccharides) of the flour are wholly broken down by enzymes (glycolized), which consume huge amounts of energy, and vital nutritive values of the wheat are exhausted, all for the benefit of yeast cell proliferation.

A close study of this rapid evolution and population explosion where oxidative energy has been supplanted by glycolyzed energy shows a cellular structure, both anarchic and prolific, which has been linked to cancer. In Germany today, cancer as well as wheat "allergies" are treated with a diet based on non-yeasted sourdough bread made from freshly ground flour, untreated by nitrogen trichloride (which is a bleaching gas used to remove the traces of yellow coloring in wheat flour, but it also denatures the flour, to allow a longer shelf life).

KNOWN KNOWLEDGE OF NATURAL LEAVENING

Man has known of natural leavening for at least 10,000 years, but carbon dioxide's role was not understood until the 17th century. Pasteur used the term "fermentation" in the 19th century to describe changes produced by yeast. Today this term refers to the enzyme-catalyzed, energy-yielding process in cells by which food molecules are broken down anaerobically (a function without oxygen). Enzymes occur in the soluble portion of the cytoplasm (that part of the cell between the nucleus and the limiting membrane) of most cells.

These oxidation-reduction reactions cause the loss or gain of hydrogen atoms, or electrons, and generate energy-rich, phosphate-containing compounds in all fermentation. Professor Claude Vincent, the father of bioelectronics (the Rh, or oxidation-reduction factor), has applied the oxidation-reduction reaction to bread making and reported the conclusion outlined above.

One product of naturally leavened bread fermentation is LR or racemic, lactic acid. When occurring spontaneously in its homofermentative form, it forms only racemic lactic acid - a type most beneficial to the organism.

When consumed in the form of naturally leavened bread, homemade pickles, or other naturally fermented foods, meaning without commercial levogyric L-lactic acid (which makes the bacteria and yeast grow faster). Added, it drains and eliminates all endogenic (formed and stored within the organism) and toxic lactic acid, thus preventing or relieving diseases.

THE FIFTH LOST ANCIENT SECRET

WHAT IS A TRUE SOURDOUGH LEAVENING (STARTER)

Very few people have ever eaten real sourdough bread. Sourdough is a ferment, a natural leavening, a wild yeast, the rising agent used to rise the bread. Our ancestors used it for centuries, it was the original rising agent in all bread, the forerunner to yeast which was the man-made synthetic version of leavening.

A true sourdough leavening is made from freshly milled 100% organic wheat flour (nothing removed), filtered water, and exposed to the natural airborne micro-organisms for a 7-day period, to allow it to gain the strength necessary to do its job of raising the bread and predigesting the bread mix, in order for it to better assimilate in our own body and to help neutralize and eliminate the allergic reacting phytic acid, which is common in all bread and which is one of the major causes of many intolerances and allergic reactions associated with bread today.

A facet of bread making most often overlooked by biologists and baking technicians alike lies in the drastic difference between the way yeast and sourdough affect the fermented dough and natural leavening. How the health of the consumer is damaged, whereas sourdough leaven offers several advantages.

Other ancient civilizations all knew intuitively that cereal grains, in order to digest required the kind of pre-digestion to extract all the nutrients from the grains. A true sourdough, starter made from 100% whole grain wheat flour, filtered water and wild air-borne microflora was the process they used to do that, not yeast.

5000 years ago, sourdough bread was already known to the Egyptians, but preparing and saving fermented dough dates even further back to prehistoric times.

Originally, the simple mixture of freshly ground flour and water, properly aged, was the sole leavening agent used. It was also done by reserving a small portion of moist dough from each batch as a starter for the next baking, just as it is still done today. This natural ferment alone not only raised the bread very well but enhanced its taste appeal while increasing its nutritional and keeping qualities. Thus, at the start of the: wheat civilization" a true natural leaven, not yeast, was the sole leavening ever used (since it supplied the carbon dioxide gas required for raising the bread).

Except for the infrequent use of fruit musts (fermented fruit juices), or raw unfiltered olive oil as more expedient wild yeast inoculants, this practice remained the only leavening used in bread making for centuries. As fruit and wine musts (a semi-liquid, unfiltered fermented base) were not available all year round, bakers reserved a small portion of moist dough from each batch as a starter for the next baking, just as they still do today.

Wild yeast, or multi-micro flora, is the natural air-borne spontaneous ferments seeded in a dough that is left exposed to a clean cool environment under specific conditions of moisture and temperature. They modify the various nutrients freed by milling the grain for optimum digestion and assimilation.

Lactic bacteria of the various beneficial type are found within the fertile medium, for example, B. pastorianum, BDelbruki, B Terno, and Saccharomyces such as S. Pastorianus, S. Cervisiae, and mucor-types living in pseudo mycelium (a slow algae-like life form). This type of microflora consumes little energy and multiplies quite slowly (yang). Its development duplicates the curves of human breathing and wheat germ growth. The bread is naturally enriched due to extra nutrient development provided by the beneficial enzymes and ferments.

A starter serves to transmute the raw elements of the wheat and other cereal grains into readily assimilable nutrients which greatly increase the healing and health maintenance properties of cereal grains. The combined action of the wild enzymes maintained within the fermented starter, plus the enzymes existing in the fresh ground whole flour, create heat and energy that leaven the bread harmoniously.

Only natural leaven assures an orderly breakdown of the wheat's proteins into precious amino acids. No other leavening method, yeast, baking soda, or unleavened bread will assure this still mysterious transmutation.

BEWARE OF IMPOSTOR WHITE SOURDOUGH LEAVENING (STARTER)

Most sourdough starters (leavening) prepared today are made with rancid, stale, dead, demineralized flour (the flour has not been milled fresh), and the bran and germ have been totally or partially removed from the flour and the flour has had chemicals added to preserve it. These facts make it an inferior sourdough starter (leavening), an impostor masquerading as the real deal and this is the reason very few people have ever tasted real sourdough leavening in bread.

This has the effect of making the sourdough leavening an inferior blend where the pseudo mycelium (the vegetative part of the thallus of the fungi, composed of several filaments) cannot feed on such debilitated flour and the bread tastes excessively sour, which tells us that, besides lacking the essential nutrients, it is unfavorable to the digestive process. Making a true sourdough starter ensures a more effective fermentation, which allows for the total elimination of the phytic acid in the baked loaf of bread and that means no allergic reactions from eating it.

HOW TO MAKE A TRUE 7-DAY, NATURAL LEAVENED, SOURDOUGH (STARTER)

This is the ancient recipe for making any natural gluten (wheat, rye) or gluten-free (rice, millet, buckwheat) sourdough starter. Using a sourdough starter is the natural rising agent, the leavening, used by our ancestors, that makes bread rise.

We use sourdough, instead of yeast, because it is part of a traditional baking process based on the integrity of the ingredients, which unlocks the rich, life-giving minerals stored tightly within the bran coats and enables all the nutrients from the grain to be extracted. It eliminates the allergy factors associated with eating everyday bread and allows the dough to be thoroughly pre-digested through fermentation, so your digestive system doesn't have to work overtime to digest the whole-grain bread. The process is the same for all types of grains.

INGREDIENTS:

Freshly milled organic flour 250grams
Filtered water 250ml
1-liter glass jar (can be bigger if you have room in your fridge)

METHOD:

- o Add 1 cup of freshly milled organic wheat flour to a stainless-steel bowl.
- o Add 1 cup of filtered water to the flour mixture and stir. Add more water if required to make a reasonably wet mix (unlike the bread mix, which is firmer). Don't make it too sloppy though.
- o Place the total mixture in a 1-liter wide-mouthed glass jar.
- o Place cheesecloth, or muslin cloth over the mouth of the jar and seal it with an elastic band.

- Place the jar outside on a veranda or somewhere safe in the backyard under a big leafy tree and away from direct sunlight and rain.

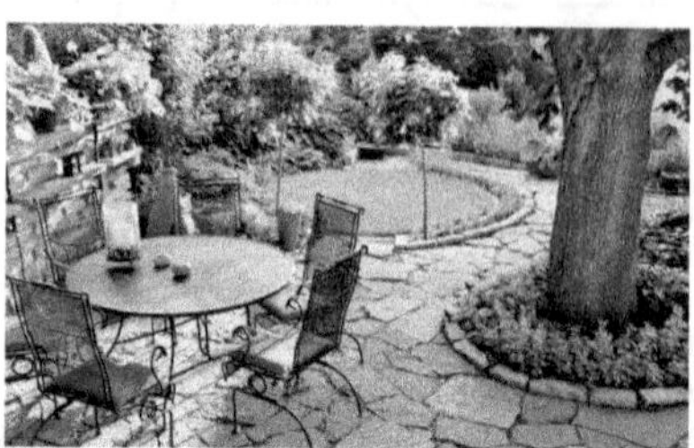

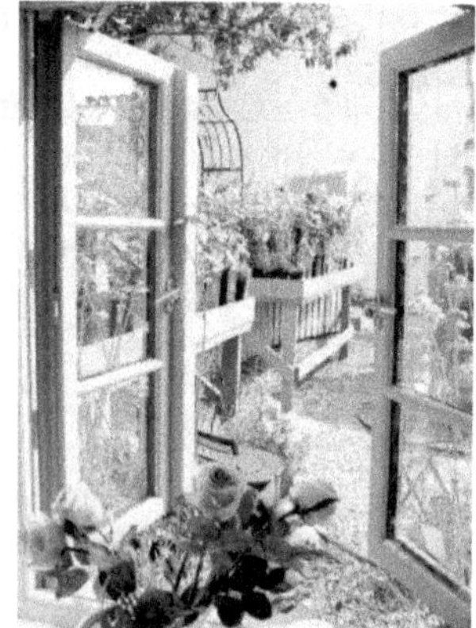

- If you live in an apartment and don't have a backyard or verandah, place the jar on an open window cell, once again away from direct sunlight and rain.

The idea of having cheesecloth to cover the mouth of the jar is to allow the airborne microorganisms to penetrate the mixture and start the fermentation process. It also protects the mixture from unwanted intruders, like cats or possums. Believe me, they love the fermented mixture.

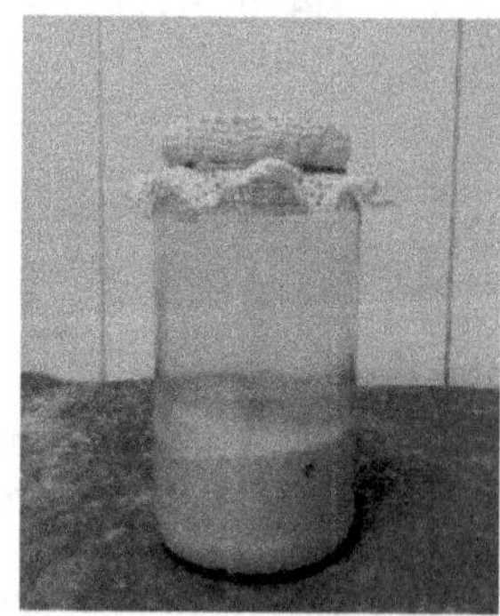

24 HOURS LATER, REPEAT THE PROCESS

- Add 1 cup of freshly milled organic wheat flour to a stainless-steel bowl.
- Add 1 cup of filtered water to the flour mixture and stir to cake mix consistency, ensuring there are no dry flour particles left in the mix.
- Then add all the mixture from the originally prepared starter the day before to the freshly made flour and water, mix, and stir to cake mix consistency.
- Thoroughly clean and dry the 1-liter jar used the previous day, pour the total finished mix into the wide-mouthed glass jar, add the cheesecloth to the top of the jar, and seal with an elastic band.
- Place the jar and contents outside in its protected area.

Repeat this procedure every 24 hours for 7 days to establish your starter, at which time the starter appears with bubbles throughout the mix. Cap the starter bottle with its original lid (not cloth) and place it in the fridge, which is where it will remain for the rest of its life.

The next day, prepare a modified sourdough starter with 250 grams of freshly milled flour, 125g of starter, and approx. 250ml of purified water, cap the starter bottle, and refrigerate it. The idea of this test run is to allow the starter to settle and build itself up slowly, so it is powerful and potent, before the big event of preparing a full batch of bread the next day. After this procedure, your starter should be ready to make up a suitable mix for bread making.

THE SIXTH LOST ANCIENT SECRET

HOW SALT CONTROLS AND IMPROVES BREAD AND OTHER FERMENTATIONS

The part salt plays in the fermentation process apply equally to brewing, miso making, the pickling of cabbage or cucumbers, or baking. It should be stated emphatically at the very start that only an unrefined salt, Celtic sea salt, blessed with all essential minerals, not merely sodium chloride, can provide the required nutritive elements. A complete salt is necessary for the harmonious proliferation of friendly bacteria. Indispensable to brew, pickle or bake a superior fermented product.

If by accident, design or ignorance, the salt is lacking, or below the required amount in bread (whether sourdough or yeast), the dough will ferment too fast and excessively. A salt-deficient dough will be too soft, slack, and sticky and the resulting loaf will be pale and lackluster. The crust won't have the characteristic attractive golden color displayed right after baking correctly salted bread. Without salt or too little salt in the dough, the crust will not form and brown well.

Excessive salt will slow down the proofing time considerably, will hold back the volume of each loaf, and prevent oven spring (the rise that occurs when placing bread in the oven). An over-salted dough will also tear easily, as it lacks strength even if gently kneaded by hand rather than by machine.

THERE ARE FIVE WAYS SALT IMPROVES FERMENTATION IN BREAD

(1) Control of dough fermentation
(2) Inhibition or checking of bacterial growth
(3) Governs, color, texture, aging
(4) Starch modification/protein enhancement
(5) Taste and digestibility

The biochemical properties of the trace elements of the Celtic light grey sea salt confer very superior results to any fermentation. Unrefined light grey Celtic sea salt, besides supplying vitally important trace minerals, contributes another appreciable quality, active bacterial life within the dough thrives on the bountiful supply of essential trace elements present in fully mineralized sea salt. Thus, the live quality of dough is enhanced spectacularly by the use of natural grey Celtic sea salt.

REFINED SALT AND FERMENTATION

Unlike table salt which contains anti-caking agents, commercial bakery salt is almost pure sodium chloride. It has been kiln-dried and totally stripped of its water complement. light grey natural sea salt contains sodium chloride in a moist crystallized form. Its water content is up to 9% which holds many of the 80-odd trace and macro minerals. Both refined and unrefined salt share a common characteristic in that both primarily contain a molecule each of sodium (Na+) and chlorine (Cl-) combined.

Once dissolved in water, however, instead of having distinct molecules of NaCl (sodium chloride) suspended in liquid, there are now separate ions, some Na+(sodium) and some Cl (chlorine) ions. Sodium and chlorine have been transformed from molecules to ions. This ionization takes place regardless of the quality of the salt used. This is an important step in understanding the process. Salt performs its job on starches, proteins, and natural sourdough leaven in its ionized form, not as a molecule.

Water, mixed in as the dough begins to form is absorbed by the proteins, starches, gluten and any other dry ingredients, such as nuts raisins, etc. This leaves no water to dissolve salt that might be added later. Bakers who use commercial salt are compelled to choose either flaked or granulated salt in order to ensure its quick dissolution. Some dilute refined salt in the water to be added to the dough. This has the drawback of slackening the just firming dough and in actuality also prevents the salt from combining easily with the now somewhat rubbery water-repellant dough.

The wall of the starter cell possesses a high-water content that is virtually salt-free. If unsalted water is added to a salted dough that has leavened, there is a natural force that strives to harmonize (balance) the two opposite sides of the wall. This force puts an osmotic pressure on the starter cell wall. The unsalted water of the cell will pass through that cell in order to dilute the dough's salt on the other side, restoring equilibrium. Having lost some of its water, the starter cell slows down its leavening action somewhat.

Conversely, excess salt in the dough creates a forceful osmotic pressure and the starter cell dehydrates rapidly. this loss of water slows down the leavening action drastically and may even stop it altogether. Most household refined salts have been treated with a water-repellant (aluminum anti-caking agent), this additive forces one to dissolve the treated table salt in a small amount of water prior to incorporating it into the dough at the beginning of the mixing, without this step the artificially created non-absorption of water will cause problems.

There is a dramatic quality improvement when unrefined natural light grey Celtic sea salt is used in bread baking. Bacterial life within the dough depends on and thrives on the proper amount of essential trace elements found only in fully mineralized sea salt. It is the same for any other living organism. Another advantage is that much less salt is required when using natural grey salt, in actuality as little as half as much.

FERMENTATION AND SALTS TRACE ELEMENTS

Proper fermentation depends upon healthy living cells proliferating within and emanating from the sourdough starter. However, unless a friendly and favorable environment is provided, these cells will neither reproduce nor survive long enough to properly inoculate the dough.

Two factors must be present to ensure a favorable climate:

(1) TEMPERATURE: start with cooled flour, cold water, and sourdough starter at a low temperature, and later, provide cool storage of the dough.

(2) SALT: It is important to use salt with the proper mineral balance (i.e., trace elements in proportion to macro minerals and correctly ionized.

Light grey Celtic sea salt is the only salt that has been scientifically validated to contain all 84 macro and micro minerals all in balanced proportions.

The semi-porous external wall or skin of the saccharomyces starter cell serves to keep its internal structure in place and allows water molecules and ionized salts to pass through in either direction of osmosis. Biologists know that refined salt prevents this osmosis from taking place while refined grey Celtic sea salt will permit the free passage of all salts.

ALTER THE TEMPERATURE WHEN

TEMPERATURE CHANGES

Outside temperature changes, barometric pressure, and moon phases, affect the leavening process. On hot days the dough ferments quicker and many times rise uncontrollably. In order to counter this, a slight increase in salt from one-tenth to three-tenths of a percent of the total dough weight will extend the dough's working time. This is called tolerance in bakery terms.

Oppositely, in winter, or whenever the temperature drops, lowering the salt level by one or two-tenths of one percent helps to keep the dough developing at the ideal pace.

Salt inhibits the proliferation of several molds and bacteria by reducing the quantity of water available for bacteria to grow on. Since bacteria cannot reproduce or feed in a reduced water site, their proliferation within the loaf is greatly hampered.

It is well to remember that natural grey Celtic sea salt contains many elements that support halophilic bacteria, which are salt-loving bacteria (halos = salt, phylic = like or thrive in). This would encourage not only the development of beneficial micro-organisms from within the loaf but also any larger organism, including humans, that elects to devour the loaf from the outside. Thus "appetence", is a quality generously provided by the use of unrefined sea salt.

Salt plays another important role to help complex carbohydrates to turn into sugars. The crust's deep color is obtained when complex sugars are turned into caramel or dextrin by a process called dextrinization, or caramelization. This process begins in the crust, since the outside of the loaf browns first as it receives the major proportion of the oven heat. Adding salt causes a lowering of the dextrinization point of any sugar, thus coloring of the crust begins earlier and turns to a more pleasing hue (color). a softer crust also results, since the crust will develop a color with much less heat required.

Naturally leavened bread is an excellent travel food, even for extended periods of extensive travel in places where naturally leavened bread is not available. Yeasted bread dries out rapidly and becomes hard and brittle in just a few hours. Naturally leavened sourdough bread, properly salted with unrefined sea salt retains its moisture for as much as a week or more. This results even without refrigeration with a minimal wrap of plain paper, or natural cellophane. plastic bags give an off taste, cause condensation, mildew, and thus poor conservation. Plastic is to be avoided as a bread packaging material, or for any fermentation.

THE SEVENTH LOST ANCIENT SECRET

RESOLVING GLUTEN ISSUES IN BREAD

The gluten that develops from the wheat protein during kneading forms into elongated strands. These strands possess positive ions on one side and negative ions on the other. Long gluten strands are needed in order to hold the dough together. Short strands can be compared with cotton staples, if these are too short, the fabric spun from them will not be durable and will tear easily. The statement "salt strengthens the gluten" must be modified to say more accurately "water makes for loose gluten strands". When water is absorbed by the proteins (glutenin, gliadin, etc.) of the flour, it creates a chain where ions of the same kind and on the same side of the strand, will repel others. Positive ions on gluten strands repel the other positive ions and on the left side, negative ions repel the other negative ions. This repelling action flattens out the kinky spirallic strand and makes for a slack or soft dough.

It is easy to spot a dough with insufficient salt, or no salt. It doesn't tighten up during the kneading and feels slacker than dough with the correct amount of salt. As soon as salt is added the $Na+$ (sodium) ions from the dissolving and ionizing salt are attracted to the negatively charged sides of the gluten strand. The Cl (chlorine) ions go to the $+$ side of the structuring gluten strand, transforming the entire strand into a more active and kinkier form.

Here every gluten strand receives a neutralizing effect from each of the sodium and chlorine ions from the salt. Each strand no longer repels the other strands as much and we obtain a tighter dough. Of course, while a tighter and stronger dough is desirable, the kneading time of a salted dough will sometimes become twice as long as an unsalted one. It requires extra kneading to render these strands more stretchy, rather than just more springy.

Our ancestors never had gluten intolerance issues in the past and if the right amount of unrefined sea salt is added to the dough at the appropriate time, tightening the gluten strand and making the bread more digestible, you won't experience gluten issues either. I do not include diagnosed coeliacs in this summary; they are gluten intolerant and require special attention; they require gluten-free bread, as gluten can cause major health problems, even death in severe cases.

Salt stiffens and hardens the protein. When it is added too early, the dough becomes hard to work and will not become elastic. This may inhibit the fermentation process or produce an uneven fermentation within the dough, yielding a loaf with a dense, heavy bottom and a lighter, open-air cell top. The resulting bread will display very large and tiny holes, a very uneven and unstable loaf.

There is a simple answer to the above dilemma. It is easy to cut down on overlong kneading time and still keep strength in the dough, add salt when the flour and water have just been combined before any kneading takes place. In this way, it will require less energy to work the dough to the desired consistency. It will thus also be possible to incorporate more liquid into the dough rendering the last loaf moister and tastier.

Maximum water absorption for the flour is a desirable goal since more water means a better taste, but it can attain this only when water is added prior to the salt. Only then do the strand's sites, either positive or negative, attract and attach water molecules to themselves before the salt ions become incorporated.

SALTS' CONTRIBUTION TO TASTE AND DIGESTIBILITY

Bread consumers invariably prefer slightly saltier bread. This preference of the taste buds is nature's automatic way of ensuring that a sufficient amount of hydrochloric acid is present within the digestive tract. Only then will the bread carbohydrates easily split and be assimilated.

Some of today's "natural" whole grain bread is made salt free, thus rendering them indigestible and inviting an acidic blood condition. White bread is over-salted in order to "borrow" a bit of flavor. Since all the bran and germ have been removed, white bread would be virtually tasteless without extra salt (up to 2½% more), sweeteners and artificial flavorings.

They design commercial mills for maximum output and heat up because of excessive speed. Thus, commercial bread lacks nutritional value and a wonderful taste as well. Salt is used to cover this flat flavor and tastelessness. Another reason for over-salting is that overripe doughs become sour, so here again, salt is used as a cover-up.

Over-salting, especially with bleached, chemicalized, refined salt, will cause disease even more readily than under-salting, or no salting. Besides, concern about the quality of salt, we always stress the vital role that the quality of the salt plays in all our staple foods, fermented as well as unfermented.

HOW MUCH SALT SHOULD I USE IN BREAD MAKING

It is important to figure the total weight of Starter + Water + Flour = Total Dough Weight, before mixing, and to get the percentage of salt to be added from the total. The average for whole wheat is between 0.8% of the total dough's weight, and up to 1.2% for spring or very light-colored wheat.

EXAMPLE: Total weight of Starter, Water & Flour = 1350 grams

The total amount of salt to be used is 0.8% of 1350 grams = 10.8 grams of Celtic sea salt.

When only the flour weight is used as a reference point for the salt dosage, the quantity of water and starter that will be added is still undefined. This inaccurate method increases the chances of error in over or under-salting.

SUMMING UP

The brewer, the baker, and the pickle maker quickly learn from experience the vital role played by the correct proportion of salt in the fermentation process. They will observe additional advantages when they switch from commercial white refined so-called salt to natural grey Celtic sea salt in the performance of the ferments. There will be an improvement in the color of the wort, dough or mash, better distribution of air cell holes, and superior taste of the product as well as better control of the entire fermentation process. In all cases, it is important to remember that when switching to natural salt, up to 50% less salt can be used.

A DAY IN THE LIFE OF A GRAIN OF WHEAT AND HOW INDUSTRIAL MILLING EFFECTS IT

In order that one has an understanding of the action of a mill on the cereal grain, and a grasp as well of the nutritional importance of the bran and germ, details of the structure of a wheat berry are given here.

Every cereal grain possesses a germ that permits the plant to reproduce itself. While only one and a half percent of the total weight of the berry, the germ contains nitrogen, fats and vitamins, highly nutritive elements which are totally transformed within two or three days of germination. These rich nutrients are altogether, delicate, and vulnerable and are lost in the separation of the germ from the flour in industrial milling and are not present in the manufacture of everyday white, wholemeal and multigrain breads.

Thus, a once very nourishing germ will be sold separately at high prices, in specialized yet worthless forms (vacuum packed, toasted) for infant, health food and convalescent formulas. Situated at one end of the berry, the germ has its own shield, but is contained within a common protective envelope, consisting of three layers.

(1) The Pericarp, or exterior layer, made of hard cellulose, which is removed in the industrial mill either by mechanical abrasion (rubbing), or by a hydraulic process. By the latter process (Steinmetz) process, this layer, which is porous for retention of the water required for germination, swells in the rapid wetting of the grain and is removed by intermittent air blasts.

We may conclude that this first layer of cellulose fiber need not absolutely be removed, for with proper prolonged soaking of the flour, as in starter, or self-leavened bread, it becomes soft enough to be harmless to the intestinal walls. By weight, this envelope represents only about 2% of the entire berry.

Steinmetz flour would be 98% extraction (pure) and this light hulling would, when done carefully by conscientious millers, yield a whole wheat with the germ intact, and retaining all of its minerals, proteins and vitamins.

(2) Directly beneath this first quite porous cellulose layer, lies another one that is hardly porous at all. This enables the grain to air dry quickly after the light hulling. This second, finer coat, is easily digested by every person and we will return to its important role, ignored by doctors, nutritionists and classical dieticians, but whose value is known to the aware, biologically orientated nutritionists.

(3) It would be very hard to remove this second layer since it is tightly bonded to the third layer, the hyaline band, which is linked to the innermost layer of protein cells. These larger cells store the essential proteins that will permit the growth of the young plant until it can synthesize its own proteins. This protein layer also contains fats, which would become rancid shortly after the grinding of the grain, due to exposure to the air. This explains why the industrial miller removes this problem layer. The hyaline band, and the protein layer, account for 10% of the total weight of the wheat berry so a 90% extraction actually removes a major part of the grain's greatest worth.

Finally, the innermost part of the grain contains the starches which are easily reduced to small and even spherical balls, passing right through the sifter, while the remaining parts, complex cells, held together by binders and hanging intricate shapes and longer fibers, will remain on top of the screen. The grain's greatest worth remains as "WASTE" and is sometimes called "refuse grain" or issues. It is this altogether starchy product that is sold as flour.

Because of the grain's complex structure, the modern roller mill does not crush the grain but proceeds with a tearing action. Rollers turning at different speeds, cause this wresting away of each coat, and when the successive sifters have removed from the starchy flour, the "refuse grain" or bran, the nutritive value of this bran retains all their valuable elements due to the impossibility of completely separating the cellulose coat of the hyaline band and the latter from the protein coat.

In a 70% extraction, we see that a full 30% of the grain is not delivered as flour. The minerals, phosphates, lipids (fats), proteins, etc. are collected and sold separately at high prices, as millers bran.

Flours that are 70%, or even 75% extraction, which represents everyday white bread, have no nutritional value. Further, we have seen earlier that these flours can no longer hold together so chemical binders are required, and extra strong leavener additives are also needed.

All of these synthetic products have a detrimental action on the human organism, and their toxic cumulative effects are now starting to be fully assessed. The reluctance of the consumer, who suspects the worst, has caused a 50-60% reduction in bread sales in the last 50 years.

This cut in bread consumption is also due to the intuitive feeling that bread no longer nourishes, that its taste is not what it used to be. Even the look of today's bread is often uninviting. Bakers are not chemists, and the amount of the various modifiers they add is not as exact as it should be. An excess will allow you to actually make a knot in a gum-like baguette, within hours after baking, and too little additive will render the breadstick hard and brittle within the same time period. While a modern loaf of everyday bread dries out excessively in a day. A wholesome whole grain bread will keep without drying out, or molding, for a full 8 days, or longer.

If it is not already evident, and what many people still ignore, is the fact that white bread is the cause of many diseases of civilization, since bread is still the base of our food supply, now ruled by chemistry, rather than ruled by biological considerations.

Just like Professor Louis Kervran did back in the early 1970s due to his publication of a 10-part series of articles "The deficiencies and unbalance of nutrition", particularly the 7th installment on mineral deficiencies resulting from the removal of the bran from the cereals. Following the publication of this part of the series, there was much interest among bread consumers, that mill designers were urged and motivated to design equipment for 98-100% extraction (pure) and starting in 1974-1975 in France and Belgium, there appeared in the large volume supermarkets, bread made with 98-100% whole grain.

We as consumers today, need to do the same thing, make a statement to bakers and supermarkets, that we don't want anymore bread made with additives of any description. Better still, go a step further and bake your own 100% whole-grain wheat sourdough bread. It is something you will not regret, and bread will never taste so good. If you can bake your own bread, you will never go hungry, it is a survival skill that will serve you and your family well for all time.

"WHY BAKE BY A PRINCIPLE"

In baking as in all circumstances, the laws of nature must be respected. It is vital if the fermented bread is to retain the dynamic character that originally developed in the wheat berry during germination.

Our breathing cycle comprises oxidation (in breadth) followed by a reduction (out breath). This same cycle is reproduced in the 5-day cycle of wheat germination. Naturally leavened bread (seeded with the wild natural leaven) exactly duplicates this cycle in the dough's rising (in breath, that corresponds to oxidation). This is followed by a reduction (out breath) during baking. This is identical to the development of the miniature seedling of wheat. Of the two methods available for leavening bread, only natural leaven follows this cycle of oxidation/reduction, which is the true cycle of life.

Oxidation is the transmutation that happens to a wheat germ cell, a live food, or an element that has been exposed to oxygen. Oxidation breaks down in the same manner that rust decomposes a nail.

Reduction is the antagonistic condition, that is gradual reduction, or absence of oxygen. It helps keep living organisms, or elements such as water, soil, or wheat in a condition that maintains their life at a higher level of harmony and strength.

Oxidation and reduction combine to create a harmonious life rhythm in all living organisms in the same way, inhaling and exhaling oxygenate the lung cells. Oxygen is increased during the in-breath and reduced on the out-breath. There is a rhythm of life at the end of the cycle of breathing in, there is a return to the beginning through exhalation in order for the cycle to repeat and our life to continue. If we continuously kept taking in oxygen, our cells would age (burn out) rapidly. Although we have been taught that deep breathing and abundant oxygen are prime requirements for good health, the out-breath (reduction) is equally important, since it allows the organism to create a void, an "empty-of-oxygen state' and thus prompts a strong need for the next cycle of oxygenation.

The study of living organisms and their oxidation-reduction cycle also allows a valid comparison between a natural cycle and an unnatural cycle. in baking yeasted bread, for instance, a strong reduction (exhalation) is followed by oxidation (inhale), leaving the bread open to rapid staling.

This is totally the opposite of the natural breathing in and breathing out the cycle of humans and of wheat germination. In natural leaven baking, oxidation occurs first in the dough; the dough goes through a reduction while baking in the oven. The crust is an effective barrier to any further oxidation, and defers aging, or staling of the baked loaf. Therefore, reduction develops a biologically balanced loaf appropriate for the organism consuming it.

"TESTING BREADS WHOLESOMENESS"

A very simple test can be carried out to determine the true acid/alkaline balance of any bread or food product. Measuring the pH, or acidity, of the internal crumb of a loaf tells us much of what we need to know about its nutritional qualities.

This acid level changes so slowly that even aged bread will test the same as fresh, providing its seeding ferment has been properly managed in storage and during its use within the raw dough, and it is baked thoroughly all the way through.

The procedure for testing is simple. Get a litmus paper strip (pHydrion) that measures from 4.9 to 6.9 in one-third of a degree increment. Cut out a small piece of the inside of the loaf and place it in a glass dish with distilled water, then stir with a glass rod until it dissolves. Dip the litmus paper in the solution and note the degree of acidity.

Natural leaven bread should show a pH of between 4 and 4.8 (ideal pH), the bread tastes sweet at this level, with only a faintly acidic taste that promotes good digestion. This condition is also evidenced by the development of regular small holes within the crumb.

The acid/alkaline test can easily detect yeast. If the bread has a pH of 4.9 to 6.5, it contains yeast, or the stock leaven has been accidentally neglected, exposed to heat(leaven is like tree moss, it dies when exposed to bright light, or excessive heat), such as that of the sun, or else the leaven has been contaminated by being stored in the proximity of beer, yeast, vinegar, cheese, miso, or any host of other antagonistic fermented substances.

HOW TO COUNTER THE RUNAWAY

DEGENERATION OF BREAD

Professor Louis Kervran, author of "breads biological transmutations" made these comments over 50 years ago. Our own Western world will soon face a dire shortage of wheat and other essential foods. Warnings of this are presently being sounded and signs are unmistakable. The famine will reduce the number of humans inhabiting this earth. This is inevitable, and it will follow three consecutive cycles.

A completion of the gradual biological degeneration that is already well underway today.

A refusal of the majority to adapt and accept, with gratitude, the basic and spartan new staples, because of their unwillingness to give up convenient and frivolous foods.

And finally, a survival of only the hardiest, or most adaptable, or those willing to forego man-made laws and once again espouse the laws of nature.

Religious and sacred records embody valuable directions for the survival of the human race. learning from these texts and practicing the directions given, therein allows our own intuition to acquire much-needed survival skills.

There is a sacred duty to point these truths out to our neighbours. Give a man a fish, feed him for a day, teach him how to fish, feed him for a lifetime. That adage or Chinese proverb applies to bread. If we give a loaf of bread that we have baked to someone, we have only assured his or her sustenance for a day. By teaching that same person to bake their own, we have assured that person and his or her kinfolk a lifetime supply of the staff of life.

STUDIES OF THE HEALTH EFFECT OF BREAD

Since bread and wheat products are such an important part of daily food consumption, it follows that such food items be healthy and wholesome. Today's milling, refining, bleaching, enriching, and additions of various chemicals to flour and baked bread cause many scientists and medical workers to question their nutritional quality as well as their safety. There is little information on what bleaching and maturing agents do to the flour other than meet baker's criteria, and toxicology tests may not realistically assess the dangers since chemicals are tested separately. The general public has become conditioned to commercial bread products and is uninformed about the effects of the quality of flour on the health of people or animals and illustrates the importance of the nutritional value of bread to physical health.

In Denmark, during World War 2, due to a food crisis, many domestic animals were slaughtered, and their grain rations were fed to humans. Consumption of white bread was stopped and replaced by bread made from whole grain of 67% rye, 21% oats, and 12% bran, called Kleiiebrot. Consequently, the death rate fell to the lowest level ever registered in Europe. There were significant declines in the incidence of high blood pressure, heart disease, kidney problems, diabetes, and cancer, and there were no cases of digestive troubles (Marine & Van Allen, 1972, Day, 1966).

In 1970, Dr. Roger Williams, of the University of Texas's, Clayton Research Foundation recorded the effects, on 64 weanling rats of being fed bread made from enriched flour. Forty were dead within ninety days, and the rest had stunted growth, whereas similar rats fed whole grain bread were normal, only three were not well.

Cereal grains and legumes play an important role in supplying nutrients, as well as over 70% of the daily energy requirements, of over two-thirds of the world's population (Edwards et al., 1971). A Nationwide (USA) Food Consumption Survey in 1977-78 found that cereal product consumption was equivalent to 226 grams of flour per day for men and 156 grams for women (Guthrie, 1989). Bread, the most common form of cereal intake in many countries has been designated the Staff of Life, and rightly so since it contains more nutrients per weight than meat, milk, potatoes, fruits, and vegetables (Thomas, 1976).

Egyptians are believed to be responsible for introducing the process of leavening around 4000 B.C. (Spicer, 1975). For a long time, bread was in fact central to their economy, as wages and bills were often paid in the form of dough (Bread Winners, 1978).

Bread may be made from various cereals, grains, and legumes. Wheat, being the oldest cereal known to man (Jenkins, 1975), is the most common. Today, wheat is the world's dominant cereal crop (Davidson & Passmore, 1986). Total world production is about 250 grams per person per day. In its unrefined state, this could supply 800 calories and 30 grams of protein per person was it evenly distributed worldwide (Davis, 1981). This amount would also supply a 25 to 49-year-old man with 30% of his energy requirements and 49% of his protein requirements (Health & Welfare, 1990). Although wheat consumption in the US decreased until the early 1970s, it has since stabilized (Pomeranz, 1988). Wheat-based foods now supply only about 20% of the daily energy requirements of US citizens but are the main source (30%) of dietary fiber in the USA (Anderson, 1985).

Wheat's pleasant flavor, long shelf-life, and unique gluten-forming characteristics (Nelson, 1985) make it the most popular grain for bread-making. Other grains used include barley, millet, oats, and rye, as well as nuts and acorns. As a result of wheat-breeding, many of the early wheat varieties, including emmer and spelt, were neglected and are little known today. Wheat breeding focused on improving both crop yield and baking qualities. In

Germany, 1000-grain weight has increased by about 40% between 1938 and 1971, resulting in a larger wheat endosperm - and therefore proportionally more starch and protein, yet less vitamins and minerals (Thomas, 1990).

Rye is a grain commonly used for bread-making in some European countries and the Soviet Union (Jenkins, 1975), partly because rye produces higher yields on poorer soils than wheat.

A fear exists among medical professionals, that emulsifiers, some of which are added to bread, may promote the absorption of otherwise non-absorbed substances, some of which may be carcinogenic. Emulsifiers include monoglycerides, diglycerides and poly compounds which usually go by variations of the words 'stearate' and 'sorb (ea., stearyl, polysorbate). Although glycerides are naturally produced by the body, this does not prove that their artificial use is safe. Some emulsifiers have been found to increase vitamin A absorption tremendously. This may be dangerous if the rest of an individual's diet supplies a large amount of vitamin A.

Enriched flour (flour where synthetic nutrients are returned, after being removed during milling) may have a lower vitamin bioavailability since synthetic vitamins have been found to act differently. For instance, they react differently to light and synthetic vitamin C does not cure scurvy in mice as quickly as natural vitamin C complex (Day 1966). Enriched flour products have also been found to lose more vitamins due to heat than non-enriched products. This is believed to be due to the absence of naturally occurring stabilizers (Mender, 1983, Thomas, 1090) because added vitamins are less heat resistant.

Many people claim to control allergic symptoms by eliminating bleached wheat products from their diets (Marine & Van Allen, 1972). These are only a few examples to illustrate the nutritional inadequacy of refined flour products.

Are you getting a better idea of what constitutes REAL BREAD, where three ingredients only are used (flour, water & salt) and the bread is made without the use of processing aids or any other artificial additives. As opposed to what is IMPOSTER BREAD (everyday, white, wholemeal, or multigrain bread), where the bran and germ have been removed from the flour, and the following ingredients have been added to the bread mix, dough conditioners, flour improvers, processing aids, chemical leavening, or any other artificial additives, it ain't real bread.

Can you see now, why, wheat, gluten, allergies, and intolerances are not the problem with bread today, but rather, herbicides, chemicals, processing aids or any other artificial additives. In addition, what is removed from the flour and added to the bread dough creates the problem, and as usual man is the instigator.

THE EIGHTH LOST ANCIENT SECRET

THE RECIPE ON HOW TO PREPARE AND BAKE REAL SOURDOUGH & ALLERGY-FREE BREAD

HOW TO PREPARE YOUR FIRST STARTER TO MAKE BREAD

When you are ready to make your loaf of bread, you can follow these steps. Depending on the size of your family, you can make up to three loaves of bread at a time and that amount should comfortably fit into your oven using a two-tier system (two loaves on the top rung of the oven and the third loaf placed in the middle of the bottom rung of the oven.

To make bread, you need to prepare a freshly made starter (leaven) to give your bread the potency to rise. Take your newly formed sourdough (the mother) starter from the fridge and place it on a bench in a warm area in your kitchen. It may take anywhere from one to three hours upwards to thaw out and be active and potent enough to be added to your new starter, that will make your bread.

If it is a warm day, you can place the starter on a window cell, exposed to sunlight. Make sure the starter has plenty of bubbles present in the mix before adding it to the new starter. That is a sign of its potency. Another sign of the starter's potency is the fact the starter inside the glass jar would have increased in size by two to three centimeters or more.

PREPARING A SOURDOUGH
STARTER FOR BREAD MAKING

This is the preparation to make up the sourdough starter you will use for making bread.

You will require a 1-litre glass jar with a lid.

- o Add 350g of freshly milled organic wheat flour to a stainless-steel bowl.
- o Add 350ml of filtered water to the flour mixture and stir. It can be a reasonably wet mix (unlike the bread mix, which is firmer). Don't make it too sloppy.
- o Add 250g of sourdough starter to the mix and stir it through to cake mix consistency.

Half-fill the contents of a glass jar with the finished mix, cap the top, and let it sit in a sunny place for 2-4 hours. Indicate on the jar with a marker pencil the point at which the jar was filled with a starter and in 2-4 hours the sourdough should have moved beyond that marked point by 4-6 centimeters if it has, it is ready to make bread. Another sign of its potency and readiness is the starter has plenty of bubbles present in the mix.

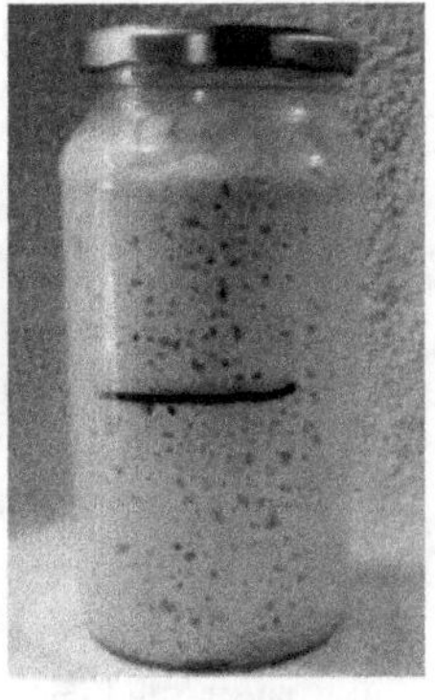

For the sake of convenience, what I usually do when making my bread starter is that I prepare it the night before. Just make up the starter as per the recipe, cap the jar, and place it in the fridge. I usually get up during the night and if it is around 2-3 am, I take the starter from the fridge and let it thaw out on the kitchen bench so when I arise at around 6 am the starter is primed and ready to go. In colder weather, I place the starter in warm (not hot) water to help with the thawing-out process.

HOW TO MAKE REAL BREAD RECIPE

METHOD:

- Mill up (grind) 650g of organic whole wheat grain flour and add to a stainless-steel bowl.
- Add 500ml of water to the mix to start with. You may require more water, so add it gradually, not all at once, until you get a cake mix consistency, (not too wet or sloppy). Make sure there are no dry particles of flour remaining prior to adding the sourdough starter. If you prepare a sloppy mixture and it happens to the best of us, don't waste the mix, just follow the rest of the directions and your loaf of bread will turn out OK, you won't be able to need the bread mix as well as you would like, and it may not be the perfect loaf, but it will still be a good edible loaf.
- You can grind up 550g of organic wheat grain flour, instead of the 650g of flour, I have mentioned in the recipe, especially if your bread tin is a little bit small, and start off adding 400ml of water, then more gradually, when required. Just remember your salt will be a lesser amount as well.
- Add 250g of the sourdough starter to the mix and stir until the starter has mixed in with the other ingredients (don't over-stir). Be sure to keep a portion of this primary starter (The Mother) for all your future baking and place the starter back in the fridge after use.
- Add 10 grams of fine Celtic sea salt just after the flour and water have been combined and before any kneading takes place. Mix the salt into the combined mixture. The total weight of my loaves is in the vicinity of 1320 grams, that is Starter + Water + Flour = 1320g, so applying 0.8% of salt to the total weight of the mixture gives a salt weight of 10 grams.

Let the combined bread mix sit in a warm place for 1-2 hours (for hygiene: cover the bowl with a clean tablecloth).

o   Grease up all sides of your bread tin with butter. I find butter works better than oil, as it allows the baked loaf, to be released from the tin, more readily. With oil, the bread tends to stick to the tin after baking.

I use a commercial bread tin, that measures, 24cm in width, 11cm in length, and 10cm deep. However, I have used a baking tin, that can be purchased from most supermarket cooking sections, the inside measurement of the tin is 24cm wide x 13cm in length wide, and 7cm deep. You can use any size tin that will accommodate the volume of your bread mixture.

o   Mill (grind) up 300 grams of freshly milled flour and place in a container. This will be used to knead the dough.
o   Add 150 grams of flour to your workbench and evenly distribute it over an area double the size of your dough mixture.

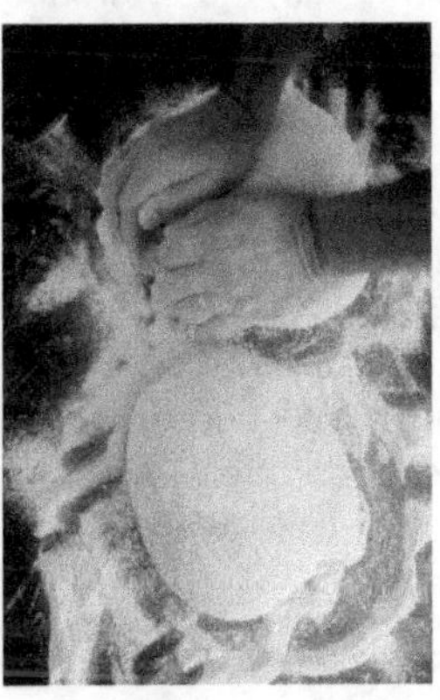

o   Take the bread dough from the bowl, place it on the workbench covered with flour, and roll it through the flour making sure the whole bread dough is covered with flour.
o   Knead your bread dough for approx. 2-3 minutes. Use the heel of the hand pressure to form the gluten. Knead until the dough is soft, fragrant, and elastic.

o   Let the mix sit for another 1-2 hours, then repeat the kneading process.
o   Shape your bread so that it fits into your bread tin. Do not fill the bread tins with dough more than 2/3 full.
o   Cut four notches across the top of the bread to cover any expansion that might occur during the baking process.
o   Place the bread tin and contents in a warm place away from the draft. Let it sit for a further 6 hours by which time it should have risen, almost to the top of the bread tin. Once in that position, it is time to commence the baking

process. Make sure your total proving time is 8 hours or more. "Proving" is the term used to explain the specific rest period from the commencement of the bread dough until it is ready to be baked. The 8-hour proving time will eliminate all phytic acid from the bread and help predigest the grain, so it is less stressful on your own digestive system when you eat it.

○ Preheat the oven to 200 degrees Fahrenheit, place a bowl of water at the bottom of the oven to supply moisture, and allow the bread to bake for 1 hour.

Good baking is knowing your oven temperature. Most ovens don't have an even distribution of heat, you will have hot and cold sections, which will impact your bread baking. You may have to adjust the temperature, usually upward to compensate for that variance.

The heat of the baking transforms all the starches into beneficial natural dextrose and enough heat must be allowed for this transmutation to happen.

○ Remove the bread from the tin, when the crust is dark brown in color and the bottom of the loaf is an even brown color and has a roasted malt fragrance, the baking is complete. Tap the bottom of the bread it should have a sharp, full echo sound. If the bread does not fit these criteria, place the bread back in the oven, minus tin and bake for a further 10 minutes, or until the bread fits the baking process conditions.

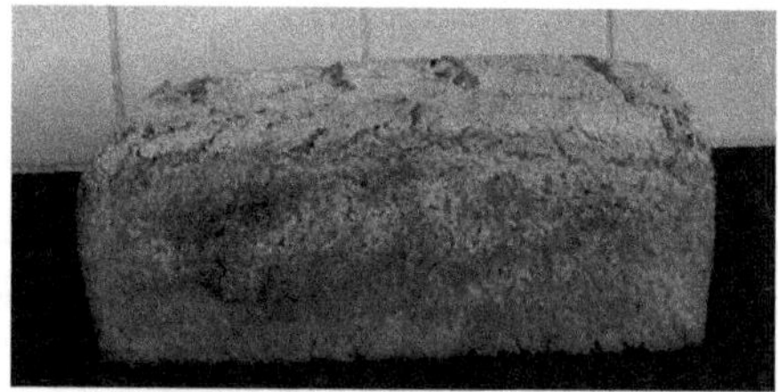

○ Place the baked bread onto a wire rack and allow it to cool in a drafty place. Opening a door and a window on opposite sides would serve this purpose. You can cool outside in a shady place as well but beware of animals and birds who just love freshly baked bread.

- A harder crust than usual is to be expected since the precious minerals have not been consumed by the yeast, and bread is a chewing food.
- Once the bread has cooled down it is ready to eat, usually, allow 4-6 hours. Sourdough bread is at its best nutritionally, 24-48 hours after baking. The temptation will be to eat the freshly baked loaf as soon as possible, so go ahead and experience warm bread and butter (yum). Try and allow at least 45-60 minutes of cooling if you want this experience. Buy yourself a sturdy bread knife.
- The bread should not be pre-sliced as the crust is its natural protection.

The best wrapping for sourdough bread is a white-glazed paper bag or wrap in a tea towel. Do not use plastic bags as this tends to suffocate the live bread.

In cooler weather, the bread can last 7 days unrefrigerated and wrapped in a tea towel or paper bag. You can leave it in the refrigerator where it will last up to 14 days. If the bread starts to get hard, warm it up in the toaster before eating. Sourdough responds to heat and once warmed, it is, as if the bread has just been baked. I like my bread warmed on every occasion, whether it's hard or soft, to experience that just-baked taste.

If you won't finish eating the bread within a month period, then, by all means, slice it up and freeze it, and even though it won't taste like a freshly baked loaf, it will still taste much better than what any other bread can offer.

Chewed along with a meal, real bread allows the food (vegetables, proteins, beans, etc.) to better digest since it supplies the needed digestive enzymes. bread also helps to harmonize the food selection of each meal.

No one will make bread as well as you. When you put your love and joy into the production of your own loaf of bread, you get the satisfaction of learning a survival skill that will last you and your family a lifetime, as well as experiencing the taste of a real healthy loaf of bread, that will satisfy your appetite from one meal to the next.

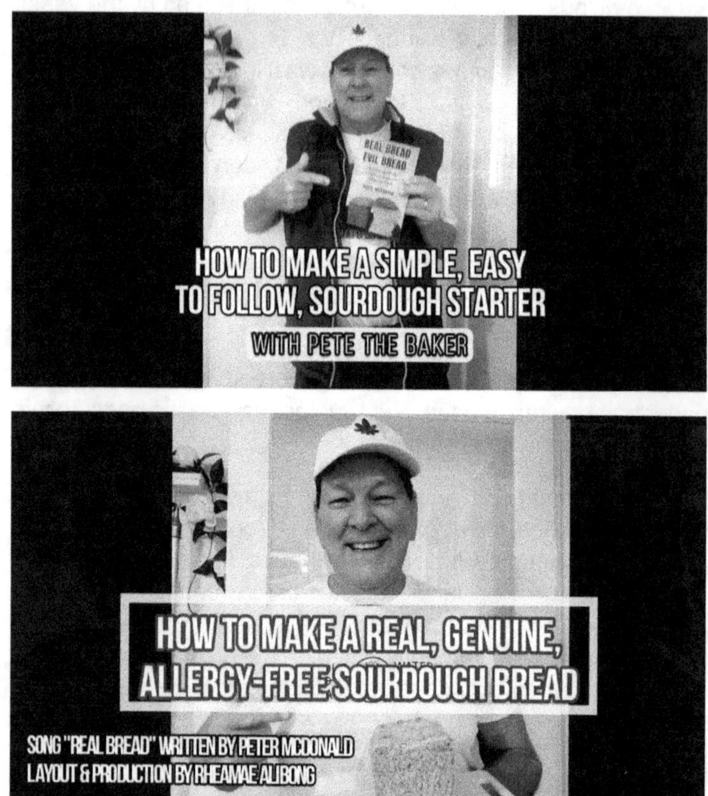

These two videos will help to illustrate and provide an extra guide, on "how to make a simple, easy to follow, sourdough starter" and "how to make a real, genuine, allergy-free sourdough bread".

THE IMPORTANCE OF MILLING YOUR OWN GRAIN AND BAKING BREAD AT HOME

Being able to bake your own bread from start to finish is a valuable life skill that will give you the knowledge that will last a lifetime and ensure you and your family never go hungry. It will give you an unfair advantage over people who eat white or wholemeal bread and processed food.

Baking your own bread will provide you with the feeling of being a pioneer in the food industry, having discovered a secret food that few people know about, a food so nutritious and so simple and easy to prepare, you will be surprised, why the so-called experts haven't discovered it before.

The advantages of milling your own grain and baking bread at home are the only way you can safely ensure that all the ingredients present in your real bread are pure, whole, and made without the use of processing aids or any other artificial additives.

Being able to bake your own bread from start to finish, including milling the grain to make the flour, mixing and kneading the dough, and ultimately baking the bread, will provide you with a great sense of satisfaction.

Baking real bread ensures you never have to worry again about intolerance and allergies to wheat, or gluten, poor digestion, intestinal problems, bloating, weight gain, high blood sugar levels, and the list goes on.

The price of whole grains can be more economical. Whole grains last longer, they can be kept for up to 10 years without losing their nutritional benefit. That is so much longer than milled flour, whether refined or whole grain, because once grain has been milled, cracked or rolled, it stales after 3 days, it becomes rancid, stale, dead flour, past its use by date.

Home milling will provide you with the freshest flour possible, flour with a sweet and nutty flavor, vitality, and superior nutrition, compared to the everyday white, wholemeal and multi-grain bread that uses flour to make bread that is stale, dead, rancid, well past its use by date. It will ensure the grain is not genetically modified and that nothing has been removed from the flour in the form of the germ and bran, the two most nutritious parts of the flour, and that the flour has not been bleached, irradiated, and various chemicals added to it. In addition, the bread dough has not been prepared with the use of processing aids or any other artificial additives.

It would be of little advantage to secure the purest uncontaminated flour from a baker or your own home mill and then pollute it with chlorinated water, iodized, or white & pink salt, or by the addition of yeast for artificially produced fermentation.

CHOOSING A GRAIN MILL FOR HOME USE

As the use of ancient and organic whole grains becomes more popular, milling your own flour increases. It is easier to find the grains than the flour, but also, they increase flavour and nutrition when the flour is freshly milled for baking.

A grain mill is one mechanism required to crush, beat, or grind the grain into flour, or meal, and usually a range of textures from fine to coarse is most desirable.

Considerations when choosing a mill include:

- The power source, manual or electric;
- Type of milling mechanism, grain mill, stand mixer, high-powered blender;
- Convenience;
- The heat produced through milling;
- Flour needed to mill, dry or oily, wet, or a combination;
- Cost of the machine;
  How often will you use it?

Once you clearly understand your requirements, selecting the features you'd like is a much simpler process.

There are mills that can be powered either manually or with electricity. Manual mills are for the energetic person because grinding by hand is a workout. The speed of milling is slower so there is little chance of heat buildup, which could damage nutrient content. If you have a lot of power outages, this may be a better choice.

The manual mills attach to a countertop or solid surface like a pasta machine or meat grinder and have a handle to turn. Some can be converted to a pulley system and powered by a stationary bicycle.

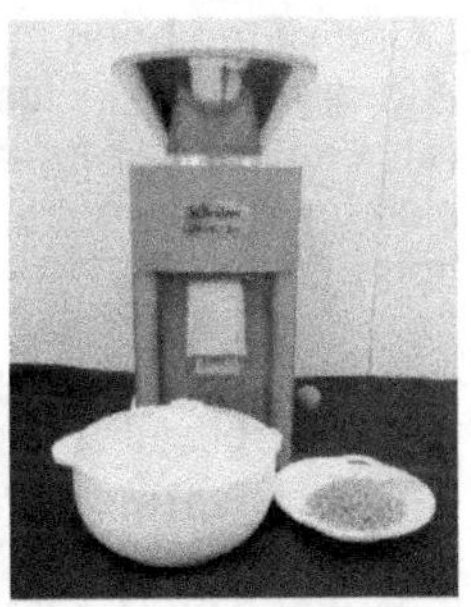

Electric mills are simple to use with a press of a button. Most machines will have a recommended list of grains they will grind. Most do not recommend grinding oily or wet items such as nuts and flax. Oat (grouts) or kernels will not grind finely in an electric stone mill, they are a moist grain and will clog up the stone. It will grind finely if rice is added on a 50/50 basis. If you require oat porridge, oat groats will grind coarsely on their own to produce that consistency.

The amount of money you spend is directly related to how frequently you plan to use the mill. Prices range from $290 upwards for manual hand mills and from $600.00 to $1,000 or more for electric mills.

Soft grains like red fife grind much faster than hard grains like Kamut and spelt. The harder grains will take longer to grind and cause concern for heat buildup.

Larger quantities milled at one time will also raise concerns about heat buildup.

One important note is that you will have whole-grain flour. They enrich most supermarket flour with the bran and germ removed. These two parts are nutritious and crucial to better health.

The wheat germ oil will go rancid, so it is better if wheat flour is milled just before use.

Making a choice requires defining your needs and doing the research. Think about how much flour you mill. If you are baking 3 loaves of bread per week, and biscuits and cakes which require the milling of at least 3 kg of grain per week, then the electric mill is the way to go. The hand mill may sound trendy and a back-to-basic approach to milling grain, but after three months the novelty can wear off.

and a back-to-basic approach to milling grain, but after three months the novelty can wear off.

One of the hand mill's real benefits is, it grinds both oily items and dry grains including wheat, rice, and other small grains. It will also grind legumes and beans as large as garbanzos. It will also grind oily seeds, nuts, herbs, and coffee with stainless steel burrs.

I used a Samap 1 hp stone ground mill for 15 years when I was teaching bread baking. I used two 1hp Samap mills when I started up my bakery. I used them whilst waiting for my commercial mill to arrive. They produced tonnes of flour during that period and never missed a beat. They are a quality mill, don't overheat easily and are very reliable in terms of not breaking down.

I did use a Samap hand mill for demonstration during my bread baking course. The hand mill does come in handy for grinding dried herbs, including sesame seeds as I made up a lot of gomasio during that period.

I have used the same Schnitzer grano 200, 600w electric mill for the last 17 years, for my home baking. I have changed the stones twice in that period and it has been very reliable for all my baking needs.

Grain mills are the first choice for obtaining the most nutritious flour for baking and is something you should aim to purchase when money permits. However, to start your journey you may need to improvise and use whatever gadget you have at your disposal right now like, stand mixers, with grinding attachments, food processors and high-powered blenders, and for that reason I mention them, as they will do the job of grinding the grain into fresh whole grain rancid free flour, with no chemicals being added to preserve it.

MIXERS

- o Stand mixers (also known as food mixers or kitchen machines) are built for baking tasks. They have a larger capacity than a food processor, so you can bake bigger batches, too. Kneading, mixing and whisking are their key strengths, but some come with extra attachments for grinding grains, blending, grating, slicing and mincing food.

o   A$100.00 to A$1050.00, although they typically cost around A$350.00.

FOOD PROCESSORS

o   Food processors can grind wheat kernels to a certain extent but will leave you with a very coarse grain and may burn out. Food processors are in your life to chop, carrots, onions, etc., not to grind hard grain.

BLENDERS

o   You can turn any seeds, berries, and grains into powders and flours with high-end blenders. High-performance blenders have high-speed motors and stainless-steel blade designs which allow grains and seeds to get ground up into flour and powder quickly and effectively.

Grains and seeds that can be ground including:

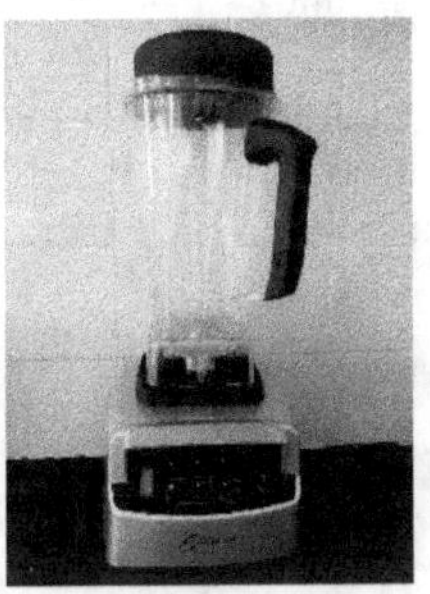

o   Coffee beans = Coffee powder
o   Wheat Berries = wheat flour
o   Oats = Oat flour
o   Flax seed = Flax meal
o   Chia seeds = Chia powder
o   Rice = Rice flour
o   Corn Kernels = Corn meal, or corn flour

Blenders can prepare a large variety of foods, including whole juices, smoothie desserts, dips, salsas, sauces, soups, nut milk, and grinding grains for flour. Prices can range from A$100.00 for a basic blender and from A$250.00 up to $700.00 for a top-of-the-range high-speed blender, which would be a requirement for the constant milling of grain for baking bread and cakes.

The biggest problem with blenders, mixers, and food processors is, they heat up if any quantity of grain is milled. This has the effect of killing the enzymes in the flour, which results in an inferior product. With constant use, the motor may burn out faster than a specific grain mill grinding machine, which translates into more costs, if this happens every couple of years. The grain mill will last anywhere from 10 to 20 years and is built to keep the grain as cool as possible during milling, so they don't spoil.

MYTHS LIES AND FALLACIES ABOUT REAL BREAD

May I make it perfectly clear, the bread I am discussing in this section and right throughout this book is real bread, that's, 100% organic whole wheat grain sourdough bread. The flour that makes the bread has been, freshly milled on the baker's premises and used immediately to make bread, nothing removed from the mix (the bran & germ), and the bread has been made without the use of processing aids or any other artificial additives.

It's the same bread our ancestors ate, bread made from three ingredients, wheat, water and salt, which was baked to a principle and a traditional baking process.

I am not talking about everyday white, wholemeal, multigrain bread, we call them, evil bread, impostor bread masquerading as real bread and continued eating of that bread will lead to allergic reactions and long-term health issues. Follow the same bread-baking principle our ancestors used and say goodbye to allergies from eating bread.

Question

BREAD AND CARBOHYDRATES SPIKE INSULIN LEVELS

Answer

IT'S A FALLACY

When I grew up in the 1950s and '60s, bread was a staple food with every meal, breakfast, lunch, and dinner. Diabetes was hardly known, and bread spiking insulin levels certainly wasn't a health issue then and if real bread is eaten, it won't be a problem today.

Bread and carbohydrates don't spike insulin levels, according to research by world authorities on real bread, and not according to our ancestors who never had a problem with high sugar levels.

These organizations certainly didn't say that bread and carbohydrates spike insulin levels:

- o   The European Association for the Study of Diabetes
- o   The Canadian Diabetes Association
- o   The Dietitians Association of Australia

All three organizations recommend high-fiber, low-GI foods for individuals with diabetes as a means of improving postprandial glycemia and weight control.

Real bread (a slow-releasing complex carbohydrate) helps to prevent type 2 diabetes from happening in the first place and manage and remove the problem (with a proper diet) for those with the problem.

The University of Sydney, Australia, has done the research for Diabetics Australia for the last 30 years. Professor Jennie Brand-Miller and her team of researchers have found that carbohydrates (bread) stimulate the secretion of insulin more than any other component of food. The slow absorption of carbohydrates in our food means that the pancreas doesn't have to work so hard and produces less insulin. If the pancreas is overstimulated over a long period of time, it may become exhausted and type 2 diabetes develops in genetically susceptible individuals.

We need to understand, the more help the pancreas gets from outside sources (medically prescribed insulin) the lazier it gets, the more dependent it is on medically prescribed insulin, and the less chance it has of a natural recovery.

Normally blood glucose levels increase slightly after eating, so if low GI food (100% organic whole grain sourdough bread GI 51) is eaten during a meal, it restricts blood sugar levels from increasing, which is certainly contrary to what the so-called spin doctors and degree ideologists are saying. Makes you wonder what source they got their information from.

A postprandial glucose test is a blood test that determines the amount of a type of sugar, called glucose in the blood after a meal.

Glucose comes from carbohydrate foods. It is the main source of energy used by the body. Normally, blood glucose levels increase slightly after eating.

Diets high in complex carbohydrates such as whole cereal grains, legumes, and Units and vegetables are usually the custom in populations with very low incidences of cardiovascular disease (Brown et al.,1985).

Studies indicate that high-fiber diets decrease blood pressure in normal as well as hypertensive subjects (Birdsall, 1985).

Diabetics, today, aren't so much troubled by, and they rarely die now of metabolic crises (hyperglycemia, or sugar in the blood) (Dr. Broda O Barnes).

The world famed, Joslin Clinic of Boston reported 46.5 percent of deaths in diabetics are due to atherosclerotic heart disease, and as many as 77 percent of deaths in diabetics are due to blood vessel disease of one type or another.

For elevated blood serum lipids, dietary recommendations include increasing carbohydrate consumption to make up 65 percent of total daily calories, emphasizing complex carbohydrates from nature, sources (Gotto et al.,1984).

Complex carbohydrates influence the absorption of fat-soluble substances from the digestive tract, and the re-absorption of bile acids and neutral steroils (Hodges et al.,1985). These recommendations are given to diabetics as well since cardiovascular disease is their most likely cause of death (Anderson et al., 1990).

A diet rich in complex carbohydrates also improves glucose metabolism in diabetic subjects, by increasing their sensitivity to insulin, therefore resulting in reduced dosage requirements (Birdsall, 1985).

In a study, Finnish wholemeal rye bread (100% wholemeal rye flour) was found to induce slower postprandial blood glucose responses in insulin-dependent diabetics than did mixed wholemeal bread (50% wholemeal rye flour & 50% white wheat flour) and white bread (100% white wheat flour). Grained wholemeal rye (35% of the wholemeal rye flour was replaced by whole rye grains) resulted in a blood glucose response similar to that after consumption of wholemeal rye bread.

In non-insulin-dependent diabetics, the differences were not statistically significant, but wholemeal rye bread produced the lowest blood glucose response. The results are believed to be due to the higher content of bran or non-digestible or non-absorbable carbohydrates in wholemeal flour, or grain (Heinonen et al., 1985). Perhaps wheat fiber's effect of reducing starch digestibility was also involved (Anderson, 1985 & Leeds, 1985).

You only have to look at empirical facts and observation which show that diabetes was a relatively unknown disease in the 1950s and 1960s when carbohydrates (bread) was a staple with every meal.

That was a period when Australians were healthy when the state of our health was so much better than it is today, when people rarely went to the doctor and antibiotics were hardly ever taken.

QUESTION

WHEAT & GLUTEN CAUSE THE ALLERGIES AND INTOLERANCE IN BREAD, REALLY?

ANSWER

AN ABSOLUTE MYTH

You hear the so-called bread experts saying week in and week out that wheat and gluten are the main culprits for allergies, intolerance, obesity, bloating, indigestion, constipation, high sugar levels, and weight gain in bread. I say that if that occurs in the bread you are eating, it is an impostor bread masquerading as real bread, it ain't real bread, it's that simple.

Let's put the record straight so there can be no more confusion. Real leavened bread as made by our ancestors for thousands of years was made with 3 ingredients, freshly milled organic flour, filtered water and Celtic sea salt, and made without the use of processing aids or any other artificial additives. Anything other than that should not be called bread.

INGREDIENTS IN REAL BREAD:

1:100% freshly milled organic whole grain wheat flour. (Today, the organic wheat kernel is kept by organic farmers and used each year for their seed. It has not been genetically modified, and no chemicals are used during the seeding, right through to the harvesting of the grain, either on the fields or on the grain. Our 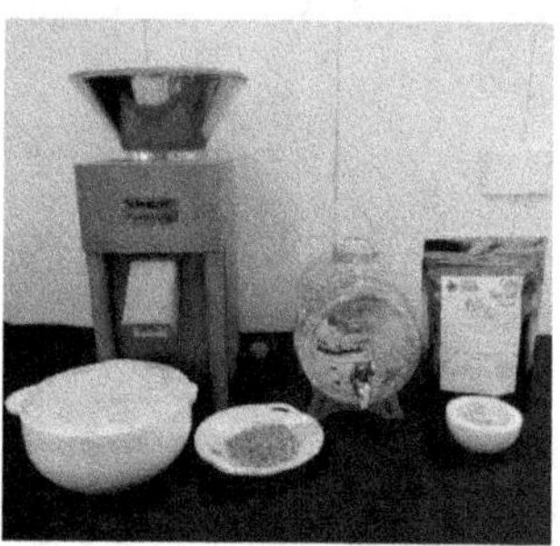 ancestors never used chemicals to grow their wheat.

2: Filtered water.

3: Natural grey sea salt. (Celtic sea salt is the only salt to be scientifically validated to contain 84 minerals).

The sourdough starter, the leavening agent that makes the bread rise before baking, is made from flour, water, and airborne microorganisms.

Nothing is removed from the flour, (The bran, germ, and starch remain intact).

Nothing is added, by that I mean, dough conditioners, flour improvers, processing aids, chemical leavening, or any other artificial additives.

Sometimes, you might not want a plain loaf - you might want it enriched or otherwise jazzed up a bit.

Additional ingredients are great as long as they are natural (e.g., seeds, nuts, cheese, milk, malt extract, herbs, oils, fats, and dried fruits) and contain no artificial additives.

THE MAIN CAUSES OF ALLERGIES IN EVERY DAY, WHITE, WHOLEMEAL, AND MULTIGRAIN BREAD

Let's look at one of the main causes of allergies and intolerance in your everyday non-organic, white, wholemeal and multigrain bread and I refer to chemicals, emulsifiers, processing aids, etc. When you have chemicals used to make rubber mats, chemicals, like the ones used to treat acne when you have carcinogenic chemicals, cause gastrointestinal upset, neurotoxic gas that may cause headaches, dizziness, visual disturbances, ventricular fibrillation, pulmonary edema, ataxia, convulsions, etc., present in everyday, white, wholemeal or multigrain bread, you have to start thinking that maybe the experts got it wrong, maybe it's not wheat or gluten that is the problem, rather these deadly chemicals and additives, which will upset the gut, the microbiome, almost immediately on eating this impostor bread and cause serious health issues if taken for long periods.

It is important to review the negative effects of additives. Many things are added to white patent flour, but even more, chemicals are added to supermarket whole wheat flour. This is because these dark flours are more appetizing than white flour to worms and weevils and require a larger dose of chemicals to ward off infestations from these insects. Also, wholemeal flour requires more preservatives since it still contains nutrients and oils that could cause rancidity with aging.

One should be very wary of these additives, most of them have never been adequately tested for potential toxicity, yet the consumer is lulled into feeling safe because they are labeled GRAS, or " generally recognized as safe." They are used liberally in today's commercial bread. As many as 80 different chemicals can be incorporated into a single fancy loaf and the law does not require that these be individually mentioned on the bread wrappers list of ingredients.

Preservatives are a good case in point, even a yeasted loaf of commercial bread retains a life of its own and will go on living inside the plastic casket or wrapper. A way to stop the growth of bacteria, fungus, and spores by using chemicals was devised and serves to still the microbial life before it causes cosmetic problems such as green or orange molds forming in bread, crust and crumb. These also effectively and permanently prevent human digestion of the same loaf.

According to Dr. Zach Bush, one of the few triples board-certified physicians in the USA, and a specialist in gut (microbiome) research, there was only a small number of people suffering from gluten sensitivity before 1992, that's when they started spraying roundup (glyphosate) on wheat crops. Since that time gluten sensitivity has escalated dramatically and of course, the experts blame the gluten in wheat for the problem, which is totally incorrect.

Roundup (glyphosate) is one of the culprits, if not the biggest problem, it acts as an antibiotic to kill the microbial diversity in your intestines. It causes a lack of oxygen in the gut lining. and that hypoxic injury upregulates the receptor for gliadin, which is the breakdown product of gluten, which then causes permeability (leaking) of the gut lining. You are not, wheat, or gluten intolerant, you are roundup (glyphosate) intolerant.

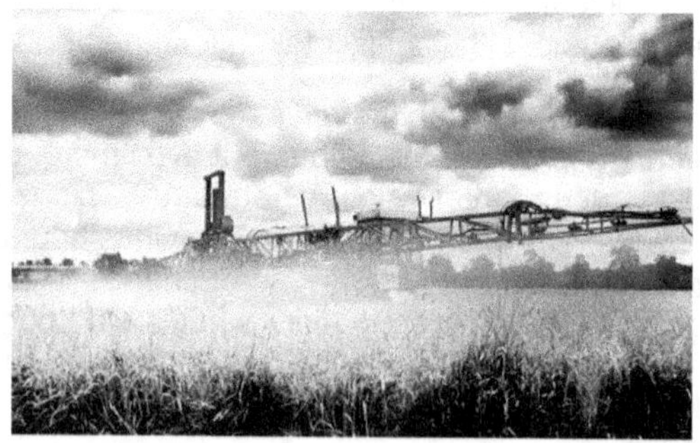

Some of the symptoms of eating food with traces of roundup (glyphosate) in them include wheat or gluten intolerance, allergies, poor digestion, intestinal problems, IBS, leaky gut, bloating, saliva, burns in the mouth and throat, nausea, vomiting, and diarrhea.

Glyphosate is the active ingredient in the popular weed killer RoundUp, and about 500 other herbicide products, exposure to Roundup, the world's most widely used herbicide, may potentially cause non-Hodgkin lymphoma. In some studies Glyphosate, the chemical in Roundup has also been linked to other health problems. These include Liver damage, Diabetes, Kidney disease, Parkinson's disease, Breathing problems, Lou Gehrig's disease, and Sterility in men.

So if you eat real bread, cereals, biscuits, cakes, and pasta, made with organic ingredients that are organic, glyphosate free and the bread is baked by traditional means, you should not have, wheat, gluten, allergy and intolerance problems. Conversely, if you are eating non-organic, everyday, white, wholemeal, or multigrain bread, biscuits. cakes, breakfast cereals, and pasta, which have been sprayed with roundup, glyphosate will be present in those foods you are eating.

Some of the toxic chemicals present in everyday, white, wholemeal, and multigrain bread include mercurials:

- **Methyl bromide** - a neurotoxic gas that may cause headaches, dizziness, visual disturbances, ventricular fibrillation, pulmonary edema, ataxia, convulsions, coma, and death.
- **Chlorine dioxide gas** - can irritate the nose and throat causing coughing and wheezing. * Breathing chlorine dioxide can irritate the lungs causing coughing and/or shortness of breath.
- **Nitrogen trichloride** - can affect you when breathed in. * Contact may irritate the skin and eyes. * High levels can interfere with the ability of the blood to carry oxygen causing headache, fatigue, dizziness, and blue color to the skin and lips.

These last two Chlorine dioxide gas and Nitrogen trichlorides are used to bleach "age", condition and preserve the sterility of the flour.

Whiteners include:

- **Alum** - the rare side effects are a feeling of throat tightness; a shallow ulcer on the skin; a significant type of allergic reaction called anaphylaxis; a skin ulcer; an allergic reaction to a drug; burns; fainting; fluid accumulation around the eye.
- **Chalk** - according to the U.S. National Library of Medicine, swallowing large quantities of chalk can cause abdominal pain, constipation, diarrhea, nausea, vomiting, and also shortness of breath, and coughing. Eating chalk should not kill you, because it's not toxic, but it's not safe.
- **Ammonium carbonate** - short-term exposure: Contact can irritate eyes and nose. Breathing ammonium carbonate can irritate the nose, throat, and lungs, causing a cough and difficulty breathing. Long-term exposure: may cause lung problems.
- **Nitrogen peroxide** - excessive sweating, shivering, nausea, vomiting, dizziness, and fatigue.

"Aged flour" is a euphemistic term employed by the milling trade to describe their old "fossilized" and depleted flour. propaganda aimed at bakers infers that, for them, aged flour works best. Aging is a catalyst for oxidation, however, and it destroys all vitamins and enzymes.

When these elements are gone, only the calories remain. In order to compensate for this flagrant deficiency, the US government has made the enriching process mandatory. To "protect" and "help" the consumer, synthetic vitamins, such as Thiamine, riboflavin, and niacin, must be added along with iron. Flour enrichment implies a loss of nutrients and should not be equated with wholesomeness. Its consumption clearly places the body at a disadvantage, casting a burden on the rest of the diet.

Considering how little is known about the absorption of iron and niacin fortification well above the level nature intended, constitutes an unproven nutritional experiment of unprecedented scale.

Most bakers and all bread and pasta factories around the world add even more chemicals during the mixing of the dough. Some of these additives attempt to overcome the obvious deadliness of flour. Dyes, anti-digestants (preservatives) and plastic softeners help retard drying and staling. All of these are part of the arsenal of today's bakeries.

Chemicals likely to be found in conventional bread include:

- **Lecithin** - is likely safe for most people.
- **Mono- and diglycerides** - no harmful effects have been specifically associated with mono- or diglycerides.
- **Carrageenan** - inflammation, bloating, irritable bowel syndrome and IBD, glucose, intolerance, colon cancer, and food allergies.
- **Calcium sulfate** - stomach pain, diarrhea, or cramping may occur.
- **Calcium carbonate** - loss of appetite, constipation, gas (flatulence) nausea, vomiting, high calcium levels, low phosphate levels, and milk-alkali syndrome.
- **Dicalcium sulfate** - nausea or vomiting; decreased appetite; constipation; dry mouth or increased thirst; or increased urination.
- **Ammonium chloride** - metabolic acidosis, rash, EEG abnormalities, seizures, mental confusion, irritability, and drowsiness.
- **Potassium bromate** - has the ability to cause cancer, especially kidney cancer, and is a significant health concern.
- **Calcium bromate** - irreversible effects include renal failure and deafness.
- **Potassium iodate** - side effects metallic taste in the mouth, swollen glands, nausea, diarrhea, vomiting, stomachache, and headache.
- **Calcium peroxide** - severely irritates and may burn the skin and eyes. Exposure can irritate the eyes, nose, and throat. Prolonged exposure can damage the skin.
- **Azodicarbonamide** - can induce asthma, other respiratory symptoms, and skin sensitization in exposed workers. The chemical used to make yoga mats and white bread.
- **Sodium propionate** - skin, eye, and respiratory irritations
- **Tricalcium phosphate** - high levels of calcium can cause constipation, nausea, vomiting, stomach pain, muscle pain, weakness, and excessive urination.

- o **Monocalcium phosphate** - high phosphate levels have been linked to kidney disease, intestinal inflammation, decreased bone density, heart conditions, and even premature death.
- o **Calcium propionate** - some people are sensitive to calcium propionate and may suffer from migraine headaches.
- o **Sodium propionate** - skin, eye, and respiratory irritations
- o **Sodium diacetate** - is an eye irritant and has been placed in Toxicity Category II for this effect.
- o **Lactic acid** - burning, itching, stinging, redness, or irritation may occur.
- o **Calcium stearoyl-2-lactylate** - is a versatile, FDA-approved food additive.
- o **Lactylic stearate** - no observed adverse effect.
- o **Sodium stearyl fumarate** - most studies have reported gastrointestinal upset and skin flushing as common side effects.
- o **Succinylated monoglycerides, Ethoxylated mono- and all-glycerides** - contain small amounts of trans fats. Monoglycerides are a type of fat, and eating a lot of foods high in them may not be healthy (Marine & Van Allen, 1972).

All of these unnecessary and potentially harmful ingredients are allowed in a recipe for a food product that can still be labeled as "bread".

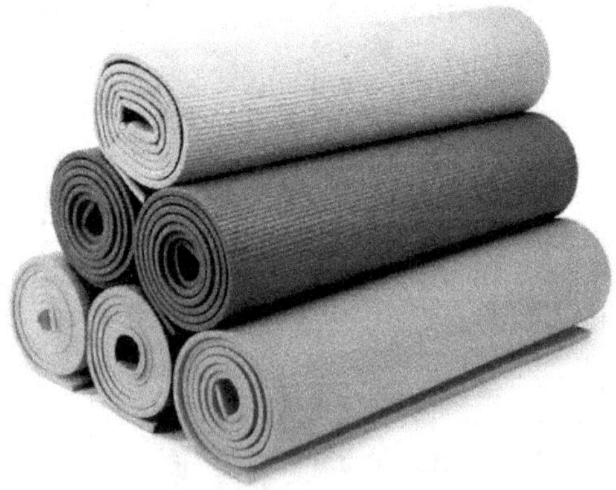

- **Azodicarbonamide** - is a dough conditioner used in bread baking, approved by U.S. Food and Drug Administration. It is the chemical, which is used to make yoga mats and shoe rubber, it causes respiratory problems and allergies. If inhaled, azodicarbonamide can cause respiratory problems.

The United States Food and Drug Administration (FDA) which is a regulatory body for the bread industry has changed the rules of nature and allowed whole grain bread to be classified as whole grain even if it has only 51% whole grain ingredients in it and the remaining 49% ingredients are white flour. When I went to school, whole meant 100%, nothing removed. You can see how easily the facts can be manipulated and the truth distorted when the rules are changed unfairly and you can see how real 100% whole wheat grain bread can be given a bad name when it has its reputation tarnished by association with an impostor bread, masquerading as real bread.

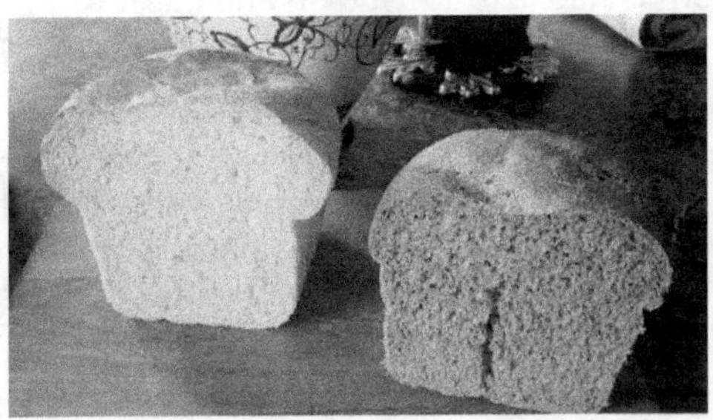

In the USA, A mixture of 51% whole grain flour and 49% white flour can be called 100% whole grain bread?????

How can food-conscious consumers counter this runaway degeneration of an important staple food? The ideal solution is to re-learn home milling and baking and follow dietary guidelines set by tradition in all the wise past civilizations. Only then are we guaranteed that no emasculation of the flour has occurred, as well as a total absence of the fast buck expedient methods that have begun to destroy the fiber of mankind.

Whole wheat bread can once again be the richest, most economical source of human energy, provided it is made with care while using the traditional natural sourdough leaven method. Bread baking must be returned to the home fire where it has always belonged. The process of making pre-biblical bread with only three ingredients, wheat, water, and salt is considerably simpler than the delicate timing of yeasted bread. It is also the only nourishing, abundantly satisfying, and waste-free baking process worth practicing.

QUESTION

BREAD CAUSES A REPETITIVE CYCLE OF CRAVINGS

ANSWER

A MYTH

Real bread's most defining characteristic that sets it apart, is the fact it satiates you better than any other food, it takes away your hunger, nutritionally fills you up and satisfies you from one meal to the next, without any allergic reaction. It satisfies your cravings and takes away the need to snack in between meals.

The proof of the pudding is always in the eating and to prove this point beyond doubt, go and eat real bread and notice how it does provide complete appetite satisfaction when you eat it, Cravings disappear and snacking in between meals stops. These qualities are what separates real bread, from your everyday impostor bread.

100% whole wheat grain sourdough bread (real bread) contains more nutrients per weight than, meat, milk, potatoes, fruits and vegetables (Thomas, 1976). It is full of nutrition and energy, it would supply a 25-49-year-old man with 30% of his energy requirements and 49% of his protein requirements (Health & Welfare, 1990).

QUESTION

THE GLYCEMIC INDEX OF WHEAT IS THE HIGHEST OF ALL FOOD

ANSWER

FALSE

Organic whole grain wheat, rye, barley, oats, corn and brown rice are low glycemic index foods, they are slow-releasing complex carbohydrates, which results in the better digestion of the food that absorbs slowly in the system and provides a gradual and relatively small blood glucose rise. Organic whole-grain wheat bread registers 51 on the glycemic index (GI), which represents a low GI food.

Many so-called bread experts have labeled whole wheat grain 72 on the glycemic index, which represents a high GI food this is a sleight of hand deception. The so-called bread experts are really talking about white bread when they refer to a 72 GI rating for bread, yet they are inferring that whole grain wheat sourdough bread has the same GI rating, so misleading.

This misleading information has led to confusion among people because some believe that whole grain bread has the same GI rating as white bread, which is incorrect, nonetheless, it cast doubts in people's minds as to whether bread in any form is good for them.

They only have to check out the "International Table of Glycemic Index and Glycemic Load" to verify the correct low GI reading for Whole grain sourdough bread, which is 51, it's that simple.

This book is aimed at correcting that error so there can be no doubt in people's minds, that real bread is a low GI food and a much superior bread than white, wholemeal or multigrain bread.

QUESTION

WHEAT BREAD CAUSES WEIGHT GAIN

ANSWER

FALSE

Whole wheat grain bread is a complex carbohydrate, with a low GI rating. Whole wheat grain does not cause weight gain in fact it produces muscle not fat. Every day, white, wholemeal and multigrain bread are simple carbohydrates, that will create weight gain because the amount of magnesium is out of balance and contains 7 times less magnesium than 98-100% whole grain bread.

Nature has compounded a sufficient quantity of magnesium to maintain biological harmony, whole wheat grain has those criteria, and the fiber present in whole grains is good for a regular bowel movement, elimination which promotes weight loss. Whereas everyday bread does not provide those criteria and the consequence of that is weight gain.

The World Health Organization's (WHO) recommendations are to eat bread several times a day. Several European countries recommend a daily bread intake of about 250g, which corresponds to 4-8 slices, depending on national food habits (World Health Organization, 2003).

Taking into account its nutritional value, real bread should constitute a vital part of the diet (in countries where bread is the major carbohydrate staple), ideally being present in all meals from breakfast to dinner. Not consuming real bread habitually contributes to an unbalanced calorie intake because the number of calories coming from foods high in fat or protein would increase, thus deviating from the recommendations for a balanced diet, where 50-55% of total calories should come from carbohydrates, 10-15% from proteins, and 30-35% from fat. Therefore, real bread should be a regular part of everybody's diet.

In one study, people on a lower-calorie diet that included whole grains, such as whole-wheat bread, lost more belly fat than those who ate only refined grains, such as white bread and white rice. Whole grains provide more vitamins, minerals, and fiber than refined ones (WebMD).

The best empirical observation, to help us realize that real bread did not contribute to weight gain is to go through your grandparent's photo albums and notice that both men and women maintained slim and streamlined builds during the 1950s and 1960s era and were healthy.

Obesity was rare in the 1950s and 1960s and yet people of that era ate hearty portions of food for their meals, such as meat and vegetables, soups, stews, and casseroles, all accompanied by bread. Bread was a staple with all meals, it helped sustain people from one meal to the next, and it was a fill-me-up food for children and adults alike. Bread was a simple food that helped the family budget and rarely was there any allergies or intolerance associated with eating it. It just shows that what they ate helped them maintain their slim and streamlined builds and bread was at the forefront in helping them in that regard.

Go do a food tolerance test with a kinesiologist to determine which food is not assimilating properly in your body. In a majority of cases, the elimination of dairy and sugar in your diet and the addition of at least one slice of real bread with every meal will see a drop in weight by as much as 8 kilograms in 3 months. It is a weight that can be maintained because you are not starving yourself, rather you can eat rather large portions of other foods for your meals.

QUESTION

CARBOHYDRATES ARE NOT ESSENTIAL FOR THE HUMAN BRAIN OR BODY

ANSWER

FALSE INFORMATION

Except during starvation, complex carbohydrates are the only source of fuel that our brains can use. The brain is the most energy-demanding of all the organs in our body, responsible for over half our obligatory energy requirements. Studies have shown that any shortfall in carbohydrate, or glucose availability has consequences for brain function.

Medical literature shows that intellectual performance is improved following the intake of a glucose load of carbohydrate-rich food. Demanding mental tasks are most improved, while easy tasks are not affected. Furthermore, blood glucose levels decline more during a period of intense cognitive processing. The tests included various measures of "intelligence" including word recall, maze learning, arithmetic, short-term memory, rapid information processing and reasoning. The improved mental ability following a carbohydrate meal was demonstrated in all types of people, young people, university students, people with diabetes, healthy elderly people and those with Alzheimer's. These new studies give us all the more reasons to avoid low carbohydrate intake.

At all times, our bodies need to maintain a minimum threshold level of glucose in the blood to serve the brain and central nervous system. If for some reason glucose levels fall below this threshold, a state called "hypoglycemia" can occur in people who take insulin. The consequences are severe, including trembling, dizziness, nausea, incoherent rambling speech and lack of coordination. If not rectified quickly, coma and death may ensue.

If we look carefully at diets all around the world, it's clear that both high and moderate intakes of carbohydrates are commensurate with good health.

QUESTION

WHEAT IS AN APPETITE STIMULANT

ANSWER

A FALLACY

Real bread is a slow-releasing complex carbohydrate and helps you maintain energy and the need to snack in between meals. It is a vital energy source, and you can't afford to leave it out of your diet. Our bodies run on fuel, just like a car runs on petrol and real bread will provide more fuel and energy, than any other food.

Real bread's most defining characteristic that sets it apart, is the fact it satiates you better than any other food, it takes away your hunger, nutritionally fills you up, and satisfies you from one meal to the next, without any allergic reaction. It satisfies your cravings and takes away the need to snack in between meals.

100% Whole wheat grain sourdough bread (real bread) contains more nutrients per weight than, meat, milk, potatoes, fruits, and vegetables" (Thomas, 1976). It is full of nutrition and energy, and it would supply a 25-49-year-old man with 30% of his energy requirements and 49% of his protein requirements" (Health & Welfare, 1990).

Question

WHEAT OR BREAD CAUSES FAT ACCUMULATION, SPECIFICALLY IN THE ABDOMEN

Answer

A MYTH

Not with real bread, and fat accumulation didn't occur with our ancestors either, they had slim and streamlined figures and wheat bread was a staple with every meal. So it is a low carbohydrate diet and poor quality saturated fat that is causing the fat accumulation around the abdomen, not wheat or bread, that is a complete myth.

When we make an effort to eat more carbohydrates, fat intake decreases, and vice versa. Foods high in carbohydrates are often bulky and filling and rich in micro-nutrients.

Our diet should consist of at least 50% carbohydrate, 30% fat, and 20% protein.

Whole wheat grain bread (carbohydrate) is the food richest in energy. No other food, meat, vegetables, or fruit can equal the nutrition and energy wheat supplies. If humanity is to be strong, its staple food must be real 100% whole wheat grain sourdough bread.

Wheaten bread was and still is our first superfood. 100% Whole wheat grain sourdough bread (real bread) contains more nutrients per weight than, meat, milk, potatoes, fruits and vegetables" (Thomas, 1976). It is full of nutrition and energy, and it would supply a 25-49-year-old man with 30% of his energy requirements and 49% of his protein requirements" (Health & Welfare, 1990).

Whole grain wheat bread is a complex carbohydrate, that provides slow-release energy, helps to delay hunger pangs, and provides fuel for working muscles long after the meal has been eaten. It is also easy on the insulin-producing cells in the pancreas. Carbohydrate (real bread) stimulates the secretion of insulin more than any other food so that the pancreas doesn't have to work so hard and produces less insulin. If the pancreas is overstimulated over a long period of time, it may become exhausted and type 2 diabetes develops in genetically susceptible individuals.

Minerals are inorganic substances required by the body in small amounts for a variety of functions. These include the formation of bones and teeth; as essential constituents of body fluids and tissues; as components of enzyme systems and for normal nerve function.

No other single food component contains all the major dietary elements (minerals) like real bread (not your everyday bread). Real bread contains seven major dietary elements (calcium, phosphorous, potassium, sulfur, sodium, chlorine, and magnesium). Other smaller quantities of trace minerals, e.g., iron, zinc, iodine, fluoride, and copper, are present in real bread and are no less important than the major trace minerals.

BREAD RECIPES

- ➤ SLIGHTLY TOASTING YOUR BREAD PRIOR TO EATING IT
- ➤ HOW TO MAKE A TRUE 7-DAY, NATURAL LEAVENED, SOURDOUGH (STARTER)
- ➤ HOW TO PREPARE AND BAKE, REAL SOURDOUGH AND ALLERGY-FREE BREAD (RECIPE)
- ➤ HOW TO MAKE SOURDOUGH FRUIT BREAD
- ➤ HOW TO MAKE PUMPKIN AND CHIVES BREAD
- ➤ HOW TO MAKE SPROUTED BREAD
- ➤ HOW TO MAKE MISO LEAVENED BREAD
- ➤ HOW TO MAKE A PIZZA OR FLATBREAD BASE
- ➤ HOW TO MAKE TRADITIONAL BREAD & BUTTER PUDDING
- ➤ HOW TO MAKE SEITAN (WHEAT MEAT)
- ➤ ANZAC BISCUIT RECIPE
- ➤ MEAL CHOICES FOR A DAY
- ➤ HEALTHY COFFEE
- ➤ POWER SMOOTHIE
- ➤ POWER PORRIDGE RECIPE
- ➤ TOASTIES RECIPE
- ➤ SARDINES ON TOAST
- ➤ AVACADOS AND BAKED BEANS ON TOAST
- ➤ CHICKEN SOUP (see recipe)
- ➤ FILIPINO PANCIT RECIPE
- ➤ MUNG BEANS & CHICKEN STEW RECIPE

RECIPES:

SLIGHTLY TOASTING SOURDOUGH BREAD PRIOR TO EATING IT

The smell and taste of eating a slice of freshly baked bread with loads of butter is heavenly. Bread is a staple food that features heavily in childhood, which is why it is one of those smells, that triggers feelings of well-being and evokes strong memories, particularly of family, childhood, and comfort.

Eating a slice of freshly baked bread still warm after baking does present some digestive issues until it has been left to cool down for at least 4-8 hours, so it is best to wait until the bread has cooled before eating it, to prevent those digestive issues happening in the first place.

For the first day, I eat a slice of the freshly baked bread, after it has cooled down, without warming it in any way. Thereafter, I warm or slightly toast a slice of bread prior to eating, because it smells and tastes just like freshly baked bread, but without digestive issues.

Slightly toasted sourdough bread with added companions, like butter with egg, or baked beans (organic of course) and Avocado, are such easy meals to prepare and they are chock full of nutrition, that will fill you up and keep you satiated for long periods, without the need to snack in between meals.

For busy working couples or families this is an ideal meal when you are under pressure, it is also great for the kids.

The idea of a good wholesome diet is one you enjoy and can sustain over a long period, that's why we choose simple meals like these because they were enjoyed in childhood, so going back to basics is not a problem for most.

RECIPES:

HOW TO MAKE A TRUE 7-DAY, NATURAL LEAVENED, SOURDOUGH (STARTER)

This is the ancient recipe for making any natural gluten (wheat, rye) or gluten-free (rice, millet, buckwheat) sourdough starter. Using a sourdough starter is the natural rising agent, the leavening, used by our ancestors, that makes bread rise.

We use sourdough, instead of yeast, because it is part of a traditional baking process based on the integrity of the ingredients, which unlocks the rich, life-giving minerals stored tightly within the bran coats and enables all the nutrients from the grain to be extracted. It eliminates the allergy factors associated with eating everyday bread and allows the dough to be thoroughly pre-digested through fermentation, so your digestive system doesn't have to work overtime to digest the whole-grain bread. The process is the same for all types of grains.

INGREDIENTS:

- Freshly milled organic flour 250grams
- Filtered water 250ml
- 1-liter glass jar (can be bigger if you have room in your fridge)

METHOD:

- Add 1 cup of freshly milled organic wheat flour to a stainless-steel bowl.
- Add 1 cup of filtered water to the flour mixture and stir. Add more water if required to make a reasonably wet mix (unlike the bread mix, which is firmer). Don't make it too sloppy though.
- Place the total mixture in a 1-liter wide-mouthed glass jar.
- Place cheesecloth, or muslin cloth over the mouth of the jar and seal it with an elastic band.

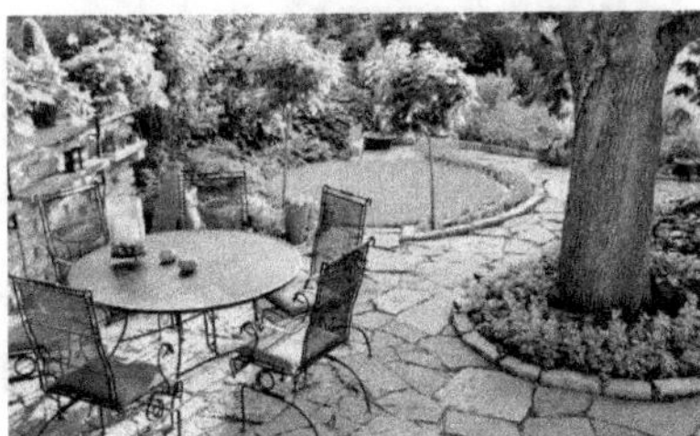

o   Place the jar outside on a veranda or somewhere safe in the backyard under a big leafy tree and away from direct sunlight and rain.

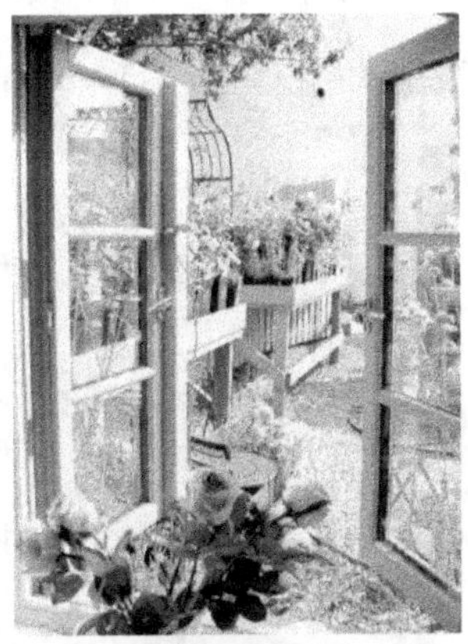

o   If you live in an apartment and don't have a backyard or verandah, place the jar on an open window cell, once again away from direct sunlight and rain.

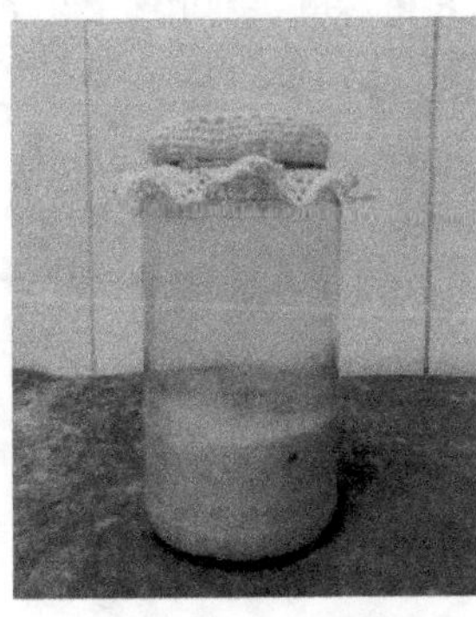

The idea of having cheesecloth to cover the mouth of the jar is to allow the airborne microorganisms to penetrate the mixture and start the fermentation process. It also protects the mixture from unwanted intruders, like cats or possums. Believe me, they love the fermented mixture.

24 HOURS LATER, REPEAT THE PROCESS:

- o Add 1 cup of freshly milled organic wheat flour to a stainless-steel bowl.
- o Add 1 cup of filtered water to the flour mixture and stir to cake mix consistency, ensuring there are no dry flour particles left in the mix.
- o Then add all the mixture from the originally prepared starter the day before to the freshly made flour and water, mix, and stir to cake mix consistency.
- o Thoroughly clean and dry the 1-liter jar used the previous day, pour the total finished mix into the wide-mouthed glass jar, add the cheesecloth to the top of the jar, and seal with an elastic band.
- o Place the jar and contents outside in its protected area.

Repeat this procedure every 24 hours for 7 days to establish your starter, at which time the starter appears with bubbles throughout the mix. Cap the starter bottle with its original lid (not cloth) and place it in the fridge, which is where it will remain for the rest of its life.

The next day, prepare a modified sourdough starter with 250 grams of freshly milled flour, 125g of starter, and approx. 250ml of purified water, cap the starter bottle, and refrigerate it. The idea of this test run is to allow the starter to settle and build itself up slowly, so it is powerful and potent, before the big event of preparing a full batch of bread the next day. After this procedure, your starter should be ready to make up a suitable mix for bread making.

RECIPES:

HOW TO PREPARE AND BAKE REAL SOURDOUGH AND ALLERGY-FREE BREAD (RECIPE)

METHOD:

- Mill up (grind) 650g of organic whole wheat grain flour and add to a stainless-steel bowl.
- Add 500ml of water to the mix to start with. You may require more water, so add it gradually, not all at once, until you get a cake mix consistency, (not too wet or sloppy). Make sure there are no dry particles of flour remaining prior to adding the sourdough starter. If you prepare a sloppy mixture and it happens to the best of us, don't waste the mix, just follow the rest of the directions and your loaf of bread will turn out OK, you won't need the bread mix as well as you would like, and it may not be the perfect loaf, but it will still be a good edible loaf.
- You can grind up 550g of organic wheat grain flour, instead of the 650g of flour, I have mentioned in the recipe, especially if your bread tin is a little bit small, and start off adding 400ml of water, then more gradually, when required. Just remember your salt will be a lesser amount as well.
- Add 250g of the sourdough starter to the mix and stir until the starter has mixed in with the other ingredients (don't over-stir). Be sure to keep a portion of this primary starter (The Mother) for all your future baking and place the starter back in the fridge after use.
- Add 10 grams of fine Celtic sea salt just after the flour and water have been combined and before any kneading takes place. Mix the salt into the combined mixture. The total weight of my loaves is in the vicinity of 1320 grams, that is Starter + Water + Flour = 1320g, so applying 0.8% of salt to the total weight of the mixture gives a salt weight of 10 grams.

Let the combined bread mix sit in a warm place for 1-2 hours (for hygiene: cover the bowl with a clean tablecloth).

- o Grease up all sides of your bread tin with butter. I find butter works better than oil, as it allows the baked loaf, to be released from the tin, more readily. With oil, the bread tends to stick to the tin after baking.

I use a commercial bread tin, that measures, 24cm in width, 11cm in length, and 10cm deep. However, I have used a baking tin, that can be purchased from most supermarket cooking sections, the inside measurement of the tin is 24cm wide x 13cm in length wide, and 7cm deep. You can use any size tin that will accommodate the volume of your bread mixture.

- o Mill (grind) up 300 grams of freshly milled flour and place in a container. This will be used to knead the dough.
- o Add 150 grams of flour to your workbench and evenly distribute it over an area double the size of your dough mixture.

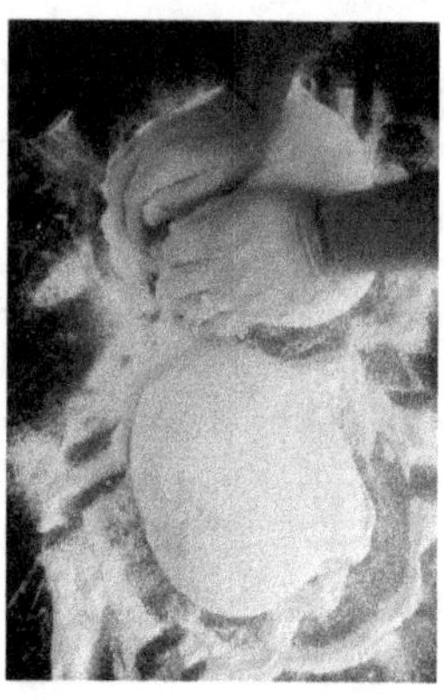

- o Take the bread dough from the bowl, place it on the workbench covered with flour, and roll it through the flour making sure the whole bread dough is covered with flour.
- o Knead your bread dough for approx. 2-3 minutes. Use the heel of the hand pressure to form the gluten. Knead until the dough is soft, fragrant, and elastic.

- o Let the mix sit for another 1-2 hours, then repeat the kneading process.
- o Shape your bread so that it fits into your bread tin. Do not fill the bread tins with dough more than 2/3 full.
- o Cut four notches across the top of the bread to cover any expansion that might occur during the baking process.

- o Place the bread tin and contents in a warm place away from the draft. Let it sit for a further 6 hours by which time it should have risen, almost to the top of the bread tin. Once in that position, it is time to commence the baking process. Make sure your total proving time is 8 hours or more. "Proving" is the term used to explain the specific rest period from the commencement of the bread dough until it is ready to be baked. The 8-hour proving time will eliminate all phytic acid from the bread and help predigest the grain, so it is less stressful on your own digestive system when you eat it.
- o Preheat the oven to 200 degrees Fahrenheit, place a bowl of water at the bottom of the oven to supply moisture, and allow the bread to bake for 1 hour.

Good baking is knowing your oven temperature. Most ovens don't have an even distribution of heat, you will have hot and cold sections, which will impact your bread baking. You may have to adjust the temperature, usually upward to compensate for that variance.

The heat of the baking transforms all the starches into beneficial natural dextrose and enough heat must be allowed for this transmutation to happen.

- o Remove the bread from the tin, when the crust is dark brown in color and the bottom of the loaf is an even brown color and has a roasted malt fragrance, the baking is complete. Tap the bottom of the bread it should have a sharp, full echo sound. If the bread does not fit these criteria, place the bread back in the oven, minus tin and bake for a further 10 minutes, or until the bread fits the baking process conditions.

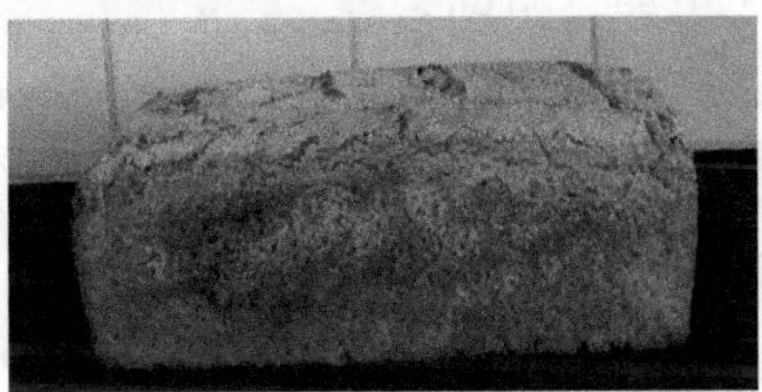

- o Place the baked bread onto a wire rack and allow it to cool in a drafty place. Opening a door and a window on opposite sides would serve this purpose. You can cool outside in a shady place as well but beware of animals and birds who just love freshly baked bread.
  - o A harder crust than usual is to be expected since the precious minerals have not been consumed by the yeast, and bread is a chewing food.
- o Once the bread has cooled down it is ready to eat, usually, allow 4-6 hours. Sourdough bread is at its best nutritionally, 24-48 hours after baking. The temptation will be to eat the freshly baked loaf as soon as possible, so go ahead and experience warm bread and butter (yum). Try and allow at least 45-60 minutes of cooling if you want this experience. Buy yourself a sturdy bread knife.
- o The bread should not be pre-sliced as the crust is its natural protection.

The best wrapping for sourdough bread is a white-glazed paper bag or wrap in a tea towel. Do not use plastic bags as this tends to suffocate the live bread.

In cooler weather, the bread can last 7 days unrefrigerated and wrapped in a tea towel or paper bag. You can leave it in the refrigerator where it will last up to 14 days. If the bread starts to get hard, warm it up in the toaster before eating. Sourdough responds to heat and once warmed, it is, as if the bread has just been baked. I like my bread warmed on every occasion, whether it's hard or soft, to experience that just-baked taste.

If you won't finish eating the bread within a month period, then, by all means, slice it up and freeze it, and even though it won't taste like a freshly baked loaf, it will still taste much better than what any other bread can offer.

Chewed along with a meal, real bread allows the food (vegetables, proteins, beans, etc.) to better digest since it supplies the needed digestive enzymes. bread also helps to harmonize the food selection of each meal.

No one will make bread as well as you. When you put your love and joy into the production of your own loaf of bread, you get the satisfaction of learning a survival skill that will last you and your family a lifetime, as well as experiencing the taste of a real healthy loaf of bread, that will satisfy your appetite from one meal to the next.

RECIPES:

HOW TO MAKE SOURDOUGH FRUIT BREAD

The sourdough fruit bread is prepared in exactly the same way

as the whole-grain wheat bread. The difference is you have added fruit to the bread mix, and you may need to prove (rest the bread) for more than 8 hours, to allow it to rise 2/3 of the height in the tin, otherwise, it will be a very dense bread.

Servings: *1 large loaf*

Ingredients:
- 550g freshly milled whole grain wheat flour
- 200g organic raisins
- 1/2 tbsp cinnamon
- 1/2 tbsp ginger
- 300g sourdough starter
- 16g Celtic sea salt
  The salt content is based on 8% of the total weight of the flour, water, soaked fruit, and sourdough starter, which comes to approx. 2019g in weight, so 8% of that amount = 16g.
- 400 ml of filtered water

Soaking the fruit in warm water for 1/2 hour, allows it to soften, become more manageable and break down more readily in the mix.

METHOD:

- Mill up (grind) 550g of organic whole wheat grain flour and add to a stainless-steel bowl.
- Add cinnamon and ginger to the dry flour and mix well.
- Add 400mls of water to the mix to start with, and add more water, gradually, if required, until you get a cake mix consistency, (not too wet or sloppy).
- Add 300g of the sourdough starter to the mix and stir until the starter has mixed in with the other ingredients (don't over-stir).
- Add 16 grams of Celtic sea salt just after the flour and water have been combined and before any kneading takes place. Mix the salt into the combined mixture.
- Add the fruit mix to the dough and mix in well.

Let the combined bread mix sit in a warm place for 1-2 hours (for hygiene cover the bowl with a clean tablecloth).

- Mill (grind) up 300 grams of freshly milled flour and place in a container. This will be used to knead the dough.
- After the 1-2 hours rest period, the dough can be kneaded for 3-5 minutes, rest the dough for a further 30-45 minutes and knead again for 3 minutes.
- Grease up all sides of your bread tin with butter. I use a commercial bread tin, that measures, 24cm in width, 11 cm in length, and 10cm deep. However, I have used a baking tin, that can be purchased from most supermarket cooking sections, the inside measurement of the tin is 24 cm wide x13 cm in length wide, and 7 cm deep. You can use any size tin that will accommodate the volume of your bread mixture.
- Shape your bread so that it fits into your bread tin. Do not fill the bread tins with dough more than 2/3rds full.
- Cut four notches across the top of the bread to cover any expansion that might occur during the baking process.
- Place the bread tin and contents in a warm place away from the draft. Let it sit for a further 6 hours by which time it should have risen, to 2/3 the height of the bread tin.

Once in that position, it is time to commence the baking process.
Because you have added extra fruit to the bread mix, you may need to prove (rest the bread) for more than 8 hours, to allow it to rise to the 2/3 height in the tin, otherwise, it will be a very dense bread.

- o Preheat the oven to 200 degrees Celsius (392 degrees Fahrenheit), place a bowl of water at the bottom of the oven to supply moisture, and allow the bread to bake for 1 hour.
- o Remove the bread from the tin, when the crust is dark brown in color and the bottom of the loaf is an even brown color and has a roasted malt fragrance, the baking is complete. Tap the bottom of the bread it should have a sharp, full echo sound. If the bread does not fit these criteria, place the bread back in the oven, minus tin and bake for a further 10 minutes, or until the bread fits the baking process conditions.
- o Place the baked bread onto a wire rack and allow it to cool in a drafty place.

RECIPES:

HOW TO MAKE PUMPKIN AND CHIVES BREAD

I like to make this bread in a round cake tin, rather than a traditional rectangular shaped tin. When I make this bread, it takes on the feeling of a real homemade traditionally baked European bread, the chives aroma, really comes through and the taste is so appealing. Everyone likes this bread.

The sourdough starter is prepared in exactly the same way as the whole-grain wheat bread.

Because you have added extra pumpkin to the bread mix, you may need to prove (rest the bread) for more than 8 hours, to allow it to rise 2/3 of the height in the tin, otherwise, it will be a very dense bread.

Servings: *1 large loaf*

Ingredients:
- 550g freshly milled whole grain wheat flour
- 200g organic mashed pumpkin
- 4 tbsp chopped dried chives
- 300g sourdough starter
- 350 ml filtered water (add more water gradually to the mix, so it is not too wet or dry, cake mix consistency)
- 10g Celtic sea salt
  The salt content is based on 8% of the total weight of the flour, water, mashed pumpkin, and sourdough starter, which comes to approx. 1250 g in weight, so 8% of that amount = 10 g.

Boil water and add 215 g pumpkin to the pot. Cook until soft, then mash. This process will reduce the pumpkin's weight to around 200g, mashed. Let it cool down before adding it to the bread mix.

METHOD:

- o Mill up (grind) 550g of organic whole wheat grain flour and add to a stainless-steel bowl.
- o Add 350mls of water to the mix to start with, and add more water, gradually, if required, until you get a cake mix consistency, (not too wet or sloppy).
- o Add 300g of the sourdough starter to the mix and stir until the starter has mixed in with the other ingredients (don't over-stir).
- o Add the mashed pumpkin to the dough and mix in well.
- o Add 10 grams of Celtic sea salt just after the flour and water have been combined and before any kneading takes place. Mix the salt into the combined mixture.

Let the combined bread mix sit in a warm place for 1-2 hours (for hygiene cover the bowl with a clean tablecloth).

- o Mill (grind) up 300 grams of freshly milled flour and place in a container. This will be used to knead the dough with. You may need to use more flour for the kneading process because this mix is slightly wetter than a normal bread mix.
- o After the 1-2 hours rest period, the dough can be kneaded for 3-5 minutes, rest the dough for a further 30-45 minutes and knead again for 3 minutes.

I use a cake tin, that measures, 20 cm in circumference, and I cover the inside with baking paper, rather than greasing up the bottom and sides of the cake tin. This allows for an easy exit, once the bread has been baked and this way, the bread doesn't stick to the sides of the tin.

- o Shape your bread so that it fits into your cake tin. Do not fill the cake tin with dough more than 2/3rds full.
- o Cut four notches across the top of the bread to cover any expansion that might occur during the baking process.

- o Place the cake tin and contents in a warm place away from the draft. Let it sit for a further 6 hours by which time it should have risen, to 2/3 the height of the bread tin. Once in that position, it is time to commence the baking process.

Because you have added mashed pumpkin to the bread mix, you may need to prove (rest the bread) for more than 8 hours, to allow it to rise to the 2/3 height in the tin, otherwise, it will be a very dense bread.

- o Preheat the oven to 200 degrees Celsius (392 degrees Fahrenheit), place a bowl of water at the bottom of the oven to supply moisture, and allow the bread to bake for 1 hour.
- o Remove the bread from the tin, when the crust is dark brown in color and the bottom of the loaf is an even brown color. Tap the bottom of the bread it should have a sharp, full echo sound. If the bread does not fit these criteria, place the bread back in the oven, minus tin and bake for a further 10 minutes, or until the bread fits the baking process conditions.
- o Place the baked bread onto a wire rack and allow it to cool in a drafty place.

RECIPES:

HOW TO MAKE SPROUTED BREAD

For each 2lb loaf (907g) wash one and a half pounds (680g) of

good bread wheat, or 10% rye and the balance wheat. Soak the grains in often-refreshed water for 24 hours (i.e., drain and rinse regularly, every three to four hours without fail).

Allow to drain well each and every time you change the water. Use a large open mesh basket or stainless-steel sieve, or the mesh part of a couscous maker. To keep the top part of the soaking grain mixture wet, cover it with a wet cotton cloth.

As soon as tiny white spots appear on the surface of the kernal, grind 9/19th of the total soaked grains coarsely in a food mill (meat grinder type with the 1/8th of an inch perforated grill is best). The 10% of the soaked grains kept whole (unground) will be added to the dough in the final stages for texture enhancement and a nutty chewiness.

CAUTION:

Prolonging the soaking of the kernels past the white tiny spot stage will make the dough glue-like and diastatic, therefore much less digestible.

Gather the dough that comes out of the grinder and add enough water so that it can be no longer rolled. Add coarse salt crystals (not fine ground salt) at the rate of 1%per pound of dough of total dough weight, a quarter to one-third of a tablespoon per pound of dough (454g). (Using crystals like Flower of the ocean, or light grey Celtic sea salt will prevent shock to the delicate enzymes of fermentation, but the fine ground will not.)

At this point, the 10% un-ground soaked cereals re-served earlier are added and the whole is worked into a well-kneaded dough. Strive to achieve a good dough structure, by observing and judging the texture.

A clay bakeware with a cover will be best to bake these loaves. Oil the inside evenly. Use just enough of a dough volume to fill the form only 2/3 full and allow it to proof at a cool room temperature for 6-12 hours or more if needed. Best to leave the pottery lids off but cover them with an absorbent cloth and kept moist during the proofing time. When the dough ball has risen near the top, place the lid on and place the covered pottery in a cold oven, but light it immediately and set it at 325 degrees Fahrenheit (163 Celsius) and bake for about 2 hours.

Allow to cool for 30 minutes. Un-molding and place and place the loaves in a cooling draft. Wrap each loaf in a glazed paper sack, a tightly woven cloth sack, or a clear cellophane bag. Once this re-sweating is accomplished, no lactic acid taste will prevail and an excellent keeping quality achieved.

PLEASE NOTE:

The spontaneous natural leavening is created by the lengthy soaking of the grains and proofing of the loaves; therefore, it is not necessary to add any starter to the dough at any time.

It is better not to use the water from the soaking of the grains as, just like a true leaven, it can give the dough a pronounced sour taste, however, the choice is yours.

Diastatic: That which creates enzymes that convert starches into dextrin.

RECIPES:

HOW TO MAKE MISO LEAVENED BREAD

In Japan, people begin their day with a bowl of miso soup,

believed to stimulate digestion and energise the body. A traditional ingredient in Japanese and Chinese diets, miso paste is made from fermented soybeans and grains and contains millions of beneficial bacteria.

Miso is rich in essential minerals and a good source of various B vitamins, including B3 (Niacin) & B12, vitamins E, K, and folic acid. As a fermented food, miso provides the gut with beneficial bacteria that help us to stay healthy, vibrant, and happy; good gut health is known to be linked to our overall mental and physical wellness.

Miso bread is a great companion when drinking miso soup. The combination makes an ideal meal, whether it be breakfast, lunch, or dinner. If you have eaten a rather large lunch, miso soup and bread is an ideal evening snack, when a full meal is not required.

The harmonious and slow ferment of Miso (aspergillus oryzae of soybean paste) is most compatible with wheat flour and produces a delicate, light-bodied, softer-crusted, naturally sweet bread.

NOTE:

The Miso (preferably Hacho miso) you use should be the unpasteurized kind out of a bulk tub. Miso sold in plastic pouches is always sterilized. Mix the amount called for in the recipe with enough warm water to liquify, using a rigid earthenware bowl (Suribachi) and a wooden pestle to reduce the miso to a smooth paste.

If the potency and purity of the miso are not right, it will produce an uneven rise in the loaf and the baked bread could be quite dense. Rather than add more miso to the mix to make it more potent and provide a more consistent rise to the bread, (it can also provide a much stronger taste to the bread, which many people might not be able to handle) I usually add a small amount of sourdough starter to the mix to give the loaf a more consistent rise.

BASIC MISO LEAVENED BREAD RECIPE:

- o 650 gm freshly milled organic whole grain wheat flour.

Any blend of whole-grain flour will work, but a minimum of 50% of the blend should consist of whole-grain wheat flour in order to have enough gluten in the finished dough.

- o 1/5 cup of Hacho or Mugi miso
- o 2 cups (500ml) of pure filtered water
  This includes the water used to extend the miso paste. More water can be added to the mix after mixing, to give the dough the right consistency.
- o 1/4 cup Olive, or Sesame oil
- o 150g Sourdough leavening (starter)
- o 11 gm Celtic sea salt

METHODOLOGY:

- o In a large earthenware or wooden mixing bowl, place the freshly milled flour and pour in the miso/water and oil, mix in well, making sure there are no dry edges.
- o Add the sourdough to the dough and mix well.
- o Add the Celtic sea salt and mix it well.

Let the combined bread mix sit in a warm place for 1-2 hours (for hygiene cover the bowl with a clean tablecloth).

- o Grease up all sides of your bread tin with butter. I find butter works better than oil, with oil, the bread tends to stick to the tin after baking I use a bread tin that can be purchased from most supermarket cooking sections, the inside measurement of the tin is 25 cm x 13 cm wide, or a cake tin if you want a rounded bread shape but you can use any size tin that will accommodate the volume of your bread mixture.

- o Mill (grind) up 300 grams of freshly milled flour and place in a container. This will be used to knead the dough with.
- o Add 150 grams of flour to your workbench and evenly distribute it over an area double the size of your dough mixture.
- o Take the bread dough from the bowl, place it on the workbench covered with flour, and roll it through the flour making sure the whole bread dough is covered with flour.
- o Knead your bread dough for approx. 3-5 minutes. Use the heel of the hand pressure to form the gluten. knead until the dough is soft, fragrant, and elastic.
- o Let the mix sit for another 30 minutes, then repeat the kneading process again.
- o Shape your bread so that it fits into your bread tin. Do not fill the bread tins with dough more than 2/3rds full.
- o Cut four notches across the top of the bread to cover any expansion that might occur during the baking process.
- o Place the bread tin and contents in a warm place away from the draft. Let it sit for a further 6 hours by which time it should have risen, almost to the top of the bread tin. Once in that position, it is time to commence the baking process.

Make sure your total proving time is 8 hours or more. Proving is the term used to explain the specific rest period from the commencement of the bread dough until it is ready to be baked. The 8-hour proving time will eliminate all phytic acid from the bread and help predigest the bread flour, so it is less stress on your own digestive system when you eat it.

- o Preheat the oven to 200 degrees Fahrenheit, place a bowl of water at the bottom of the oven to supply moisture and allow the bread to bake for 1 hour.

Good baking is knowing your oven temperature. Most ovens don't have an even distribution of heat, you will have hot and cold sections, which will impact your bread baking. You may have to adjust the temperature, usually upward to compensate for that variance.

The heat of the baking transforms all the starches into beneficial natural dextrose and enough heat must be allowed for this transmutation to happen.

- o Remove the bread from the tin, when the crust is dark brown in color and the bottom of the loaf is an even brown color and has a roasted malt fragrance, the baking is complete. Tap the bottom of the bread it should have a sharp, full echo sound. If the bread does not fit these criteria, place the bread back in the oven, minus tin and bake for a further 10 minutes, or until the bread fits the baking process conditions.
- o Place the baked bread onto a wire rack and allow it to cool in a drafty place. Opening a door and a window on opposite sides would serve this purpose. You can cool outside in a shady place as well but beware of animals and birds who just love freshly baked bread.

A harder crust than usual is to be expected since the precious minerals have not been consumed by the yeast, and bread is a chewing food.

Once the bread has cooled down it is ready to eat, usually, allow 4-6 hours. Sourdough bread is at its best nutritionally, 24-48 hours after baking. The temptation will be to eat the freshly baked loaf as soon as possible, so go ahead and experience warm bread and butter (yum). Try and allow at least 45-60 minutes of cooling if you want this experience. Buy yourself a sturdy bread knife.

The bread should not be pre-sliced as the crust is its natural protection.

The best wrapping for sourdough bread is a white-glazed paper bag. or wrap it in a tea towel. Do not use plastic bags as this tends to suffocate the live bread.

In cooler weather, the bread can last 7 days unrefrigerated and wrapped in a tea towel or paper bag. You can leave it in the refrigerator where it will last up to 14 days. If the bread starts to get hard, warm it up in the toaster before eating. Sourdough responds to heat and once warmed it's as if the bread has just been baked. I like my bread warmed on every occasion, whether it's hard or soft, to experience that just-baked taste.

Begin kneading in a circular pattern, using the heel of the hand pressure to form the gluten. Mix about 300 times or until the dough is soft, fragrant and elastic. Add either flour or water to achieve the consistency of a fleshy earlobe.

Place the dough in a clean wooden bowl, cover it with 4 damp layers of clean unprinted, cotton toweling and allow it to mature in a draft-free place. Depending on the amount of heat present in the proofing area, the dough will mature from 2-8 hours and change taste accordingly. The longer the proofing time, the more sweet and sour will the bread be. The degree of ripeness of the dough can be followed by making a sharp cut into the dough, when very tiny air bubbles are noted, the dough is ready for baking.

RECIPES:

HOW TO MAKE A PIZZA OR FLATBREAD BASE

On baking day, try and cover your total baking requirements for the week, which can include your bread, pizza bases, cakes, etc.

When you start baking with whole wheat grain flour, and sourdough starter, for all your grain-based baking requirements, you will see and feel the difference it makes to your weight management, how satisfied you feel after every meal, and notice that there is no bloating associated with whole grain baking.

You can also use the pizza base as a form of flatbread, if you wish, instead of the customary high-loaf bread.

Sourdough organic whole wheat grain pizza

The proof is always in the eating, and this is another example of how sourdough baking satisfies your hunger. Take the simple whole-grain wheaten pizza. This is a real yummy meal and something we look forward to.

A 31 cm pizza base with all the trimmings added and divided into quarters will successfully feed a family of 4. The wonderful thing about this experience is if eaten at lunchtime you will only require a very small dinner, which might include a sandwich, or fruit because your hunger is still very much satisfied. You will notice how light you feel in the stomach after eating the pizza, which in itself is quite remarkable.

PIZZA BASE:

The ingredients are the same as for baking bread but with a smaller amount.

METHOD:

- o Mill up (grind) 300g of organic whole wheat grain flour and add to a stainless-steel bowl.
- o Add 250ml of water to the mix to start with. You may require more water, so add it gradually, not all at once, until you get a cake mix consistency, (not too wet or sloppy).
- o Add 250g of the sourdough starter to the mix and stir until the starter has mixed in with the other ingredients (don't over-stir).
- o Add 6 grams of fine Celtic sea salt just after the flour and water have been combined and before any kneading takes place. Mix the salt into the combined mixture.

Let the combined bread mix sit in a warm place for 1-2 hours (for hygiene cover the bowl with a clean tablecloth).

- o Mill (grind) up 200 grams of freshly milled flour and place in a container. This will be used to knead the dough.
- o Add 150 grams of flour to your workbench and evenly distribute it over an area double the size of your dough mixture.
- o Take the dough from the bowl, place it on the workbench covered with flour, and roll it through the flour making sure the whole dough is covered with flour.
- o Knead your pizza dough for approx. 2-3 minutes. Use the heel of the hand pressure to form the gluten. knead until the dough is soft, fragrant, and elastic.

Let the mix sit for another 1-2 hours, then repeat the kneading process again.

Grease up your pizza tray with butter. I find butter works better than oil, as it allows the baked pizza, to be released from the tray, more readily. With oil, the dough tends to stick to the tray after baking.

I use a normal pizza tray with an internal measurement of 30cm circumference.

Shape your pizza dough so that it fits onto your pizza tray, evenly.

- o Place the pizza tray and contents in a warm place away from the draft. Let it sit for a further 6 hours. It is time to commence the baking process. Make sure your total proving time is 8 hours or more. Proving is the term used to explain the specific rest period from the commencement of preparing the dough until it is ready to be baked. The 8-hour proving time will eliminate all phytic acid from the dough and help predigest the grain, so it is less stress on your own digestive system when you eat it.
- o Preheat the oven to 225 degrees Fahrenheit, place a bowl of water at the bottom of the oven to supply moisture, and allow the pizza to bake for 30 minutes.

Good baking is knowing your oven temperature. Most ovens don't have an even distribution of heat, you will have hot and cold sections, which will impact your bread baking. You may have to adjust the temperature, usually upward to compensate for that variance.

The heat of the baking transforms all the starches into beneficial natural dextrose and enough heat must be allowed for this transmutation to happen.

After 30 minutes, remove the pizza base from the tray, place the baked pizza base onto a wire rack, and allow it to cool in a drafty place. The best wrapping for the pizza base is a white glazed paper bag and leave it in the fridge until you are ready to use it. Or, if you are going to use it within 2 days after it cools down, wrap it in a tea towel and leave it on a bench. Do not use plastic bags as this tends to suffocate the live pizza base.

When you are ready to prepare your pizza, add all the ingredients and bake in the oven at 200 degrees Fahrenheit for 20 minutes. It is now ready to eat. Enjoy.

SOME PIZZA COMBINATIONS

> ## SEAFOOD PIZZA:

- Add 1/2 cup tomato paste (cover the base of the pizza).
- Evenly spread 250g canned Mackerel fillets to the base.
- Add 250g smoked oysters oysters
- Slice up 1 large tomato and garnish the top of the pizza.
- Add Celtic sea salt and cracked pepper to taste.
- Sprinkle 1 cup of grated cheese over the top of the pizza.
- Bake for 20 minutes.

> ## HAWAIIAN PIZZA:

- Add 1 cup of organic tomato sauce (cover the base of the pizza).
- 100g of sliced smoked ham (to cover the pizza base)
- 332 g canned pineapple chunks (strain off the juice) and add evenly over the base of the pizza.
- Sprinkle 1/3 tsp Celtic sea salt over the ingredients, or to taste.
- Sprinkle 1 cup of grated cheese on the top of the pizza.
- Bake for 20 minutes.

Now that's an inexpensive meal.

RECIPES:

HOW TO MAKE TRADITIONAL BREAD & BUTTER PUDDING

It brings back fond childhood memories, of dinner time with the

family. Those cold winter nights, a warm fire, meat and three vegetable dinners, and bread & butter pudding for dessert.

INGREDIENTS:

- o   5 free range, or organic eggs
- o   2 cups milk of choice (Soy, Almond, or Rice)
- o   300 ml pure cream
- o   1/4 cup coconut sugar
- o   1 teaspoon vanilla essence
- o   1/4 teaspoon ground cinnamon
- o   1/4 ground ginger
- o   8 thick slices of sourdough bread, crusts removed
- o   40g butter, softened
- o   1/2 cup sultanas
- o   1/2 teaspoon Celtic sea salt

METHOD:

Step 1
Preheat oven to 180°C/160°C fan forced. Grease a 5cm-deep, 17cm x 28cm (base) baking dish. Whisk eggs, milk, cream, coconut sugar, vanilla, ginger, salt and cinnamon in a bowl.

Step 2
Spread both sides of each bread slice with butter. Cut each slice in half diagonally. Arrange half the bread in rows in the prepared dish. Sprinkle with half the sultanas. Repeat with remaining bread and sultanas.

Step 3
Pour egg mixture over the bread. Bake for 30 to 35 minutes or until golden and set. Serve.

RECIPES:

HOW TO MAKE SEITAN
(Known as wheat meat, or mock chicken meat)

Wheat gluten has been used as a substitute for meat in Asian countries for centuries, particularly among Buddhists who prefer not to eat meat. George Ohsawa, the Japanese advocate for the "macrobiotic" diet, coined the term seitan for wheat gluten in the early 1960s. Seitan's versatility and "meatiness", combined with the need for tasty, vegan protein options have contributed to its huge increase in popularity worldwide in recent years.

As well as being flavorsome and reminiscent of meat, seitan is relatively high in protein and non-hame iron compared to other vegetarian protein foods. One serving around the size of the palm of your hand contains about 75 grams of protein, enough for most adults for a day. Gram for gram, that's about three times as much protein as beef or lamb. With about 5 milligrams of iron per 100 grams, seitan has as much iron as kangaroo meat or beef.

But as for other plant-based foods, the non-hame iron in seitan is not as readily absorbed as the hame iron in meats. A small serving of seitan (100 grams) contains about 14 grams of carbs, which is about the same as one slice of bread. Seitan doesn't contain any soy, unlike tofu or tempeh. So it's a good option.

Here is one of the most common methods to make seitan at home, using the 'wash the flour' method:

PREP TIME: 30 minutes
COOK TIME: 1 hour
TOTAL TIME: 1 hour 30 minutes

INGREDIENTS A:

- 1 kg freshly milled organic wheat flour
- filtered water

INGREDIENTS B:

- 100 ml organic coconut amino sauce or light soy sauce
- 20 ml organic coconut BBQ sauce or dark soy sauce
- 20 ml organic coconut balsamic vinegar, or dry sherry, or cooking wine
- 1 bay leaf
- 1 star anise
- 1 cinnamon bark
- 4 cloves
- 1 bay leaf
- 1 star anise
- 1 cinnamon bark
- 4 cloves

INSTRUCTIONS:

Essentially, the flour is kneaded with water to form a dough, just like making bread minus the salt.

Next, wash the dough gently with water several times until most of the starch is removed from the dough, leaving mainly the wheat protein behind.

<u>KNEAD THE DOUGH</u>

- Mix the water with the flour and knead it until it forms a non-sticky dough.
- Knead the dough for ten minutes until the surface becomes shiny, and gluten is formed.
- Submerge the dough in water for two hours.

WASH AWAY THE STARCH

o   Wash the dough for three minutes to release the starch into the water. When the water becomes milky, pour it away and use fresh water to rewash it.
o   Repeat the washing process a few times until the water becomes semi-translucent.
o   Let the washed dough rest for fifteen minutes.

BRAID THE SEITAN

o   Place the seitan on a work surface, then stretch it until it is elongated like a rod.
o   Cut the seitan lengthwise with a sharp knife into three parts, with one end attached.
o   Start to stretch and braid the gluten like making braided bread. Finally, tuck the end into the dough to close it up.
o   After that, make a few knots to tighten the gluten further.

BRAISE THE SEITAN

o   Bring ingredients B to a boil.
o   Place the seitan in braising liquid and simmer for about an hour. Add more water if necessary.
o   Transfer the seitan and the braising liquid to a ziplock bag or sealed container and refrigerate overnight.

RECIPES:

ANZAC BISCUIT RECIPE

ANZAC BISCUITS PAY TRIBUTE TO OUR SOLDIERS WHO FOUGHT FOR OUR FREEDOM.

Anzac Day is a day of remembrance observed in Australia and New Zealand. It falls on the anniversary of the Australian and New Zealand Army Corps (ANZAC) landing at Gallipoli, in Turkey. The day was originally observed to honor the soldiers who died in that conflict but now commemorates and honors all Australian and New Zealand soldiers.

During the first and second world wars, wives and women's groups would bake biscuits and send them to their husbands on the battlefield. Biscuits were a tasty treat but had to be made from ingredients that didn't spoil easily, as there was no express post (or FedEx), so everything was sent by ship.

I have made my Anzac biscuits, with some additional ingredients, that were not in the original Anzac biscuit recipe. The butter and eggs give more taste and texture to the biscuit.

INGREDIENTS:

- 1 cup freshly milled, organic, rancid-free, coarse oat flour (100g)
- 1 cup freshly milled organic whole flour (150g)
- 1 cup organic coconut sugar (220g)
- 1/2 cup organic, desiccated coconut 40g
- 250 g (4 ounces) organic butter, melted
- 2 tbsp coconut nectar
- 1 tsp organic vanilla essence
- 2 free-range eggs
- 5 g Celtic sea salt
- 250 g sourdough starter
- Egg rings, or hand shape

METHOD:

- o Preheat oven to 200°C. Grease egg rings with butter; line the tray with baking paper. add rings to the tray.
- o Combine oat & wheat, flour, sugar, and coconut in a large bowl. Place butter (melted), syrup, and vanilla essence, in a bowl, whip up the eggs and add to the wet mix. Mix thoroughly all wet mix ingredients.
- o Add sourdough starter to the mix, and stir thoroughly.
- o Add Celtic sea salt to the mix, stir thoroughly.
- o Add mixture to the egg rings, about 3/4 capacity, flatten slightly, or hand shape the mixture.
- o Let the finished product sit for 8 hours.
- o Bake for 20 minutes at 200 C or until golden; cool on trays.

All ovens are different, they have hot and cold spots within them. Make a note of the time and oven temperature that the biscuits were baked.

RECIPES:

MEAL CHOICES FOR A DAY

Breakfast

- o Reishi, or Cordyceps health coffee (see details)
- o Power porridge (see recipe)
- o A slice of toasted sourdough fruit bread and butter
- o Avocado, and baked beans on toasted sourdough bread
- o Power smoothie (see recipe)

SNACKS

- o A slice of sourdough fruit bread & butter
- o A slice of sourdough bread with peanut butter

LUNCH

- o A ham, cheese, and tomato sourdough toastie
- o Sardines, or oysters on a slice of sourdough bread

DINNER

- o Chicken soup with a slice of sourdough bread (see recipe)
- o Pancit with a slice of sourdough bread (see recipe)
- o Mung beans & chicken stew

RECIPES:
HEALTHY COFFEE

Some experts say coffee is bad for you, while others say it's fine it helps to improve mental performance, especially alertness, attention, and concentration. It is a mild stimulant and when it is infused with either of the two most powerful herbs in Chinese medicine, the Reishi mushroom and Cordyceps Sinensis mushroom, it ensures the health benefits of those herbs are sent to all parts of the body, immediately. So from that perspective, healthy coffee is a wonderful way of subtly getting health benefits to people who don't take supplements, who are suffering from fatigue, hormone imbalance, or some other health issue.

My journey with healthy coffee started in 2004 when I first discovered the health benefits of the Reishi mushroom and Cordyceps Sinensis (a fungus). My problem was, normal coffee gave me heart palpitations and stomach jitters, at that stage I had been off any caffeine drinks for 20 years, so although the idea was sound if this coffee gave me palpitations, there was no way I would drink it and to my great delight it didn't.

Reishi and Cordyceps infused coffee is energy and nutrition in a cup. If ever you feel hungry, drink a cup of either and notice how it satisfies your hunger pangs. They are ideal drinks to stop you from snacking between meals.

INGREDIENTS:

- 1tsp Instant Brazilian coffee
- 400 mg or 1 capsule Reishi mushroom or Cordyceps sinensis mushroom
- Coconut sugar, or sweetener of your choice
- Milk of choice, OR coconut milk if you want coconut coffee

DIRECTIONS:

<u>HEALTHY BLACK COFFEE</u>

- o Add 1 x tsp of Brazilian instant coffee to a cup of hot water, break open one Reishi, or Cordyceps capsule, and add to the coffee, add coconut sugar to the mix, if required, your energy in a cup is now ready to drink.

<u>HEALTHY WHITE COFFEE</u>

- o The same ingredients as with the healthy black coffee, but just add the milk of your choice to the Beveridge.

If you prefer your own percolated cappuccino or flat white coffee, just break open one Reishi, or Cordyceps capsule, and add it to your coffee.

The Reishi mushroom and Cordyceps sinensis fungus are truly amazing herbs that date back 4500 years in Chinese medicine. In Chinese folklore The Reishi mushroom was a herb only available to the Emperor or nobility under punishment of death, that is how much they revered it in those days and still do to this day. If you visit China, just ask one of the locals about Reishi or Lingzhi as it is better known there, they have nothing but praise for its health benefits, whatever that may be.

Now there is scientific validation to back up those claims, Reishi for instance as well as being an outstanding herb to balance hormones, has had more clinical trials done for cancer than anything else on the planet refer http://www.pubmed.org cancer - Reishi. Reishi is an adaptogen meaning it balances imbalance in the body whether that be high blood pressure, or high blood sugar, provides sustained energy, acts as a wonderful calmative and provides many more health benefits.

Cordyceps Sinensis is the king herb of energy, fatigue and recovery in Chinese medicine, and you only have to research the clinical data on how it improves respiratory function, including bronchitis and asthma to see why. Google, (Reference 2, Chapter "Effects on the Respiratory System", pages 429-432).

There have been over 1400 clinical trials conducted and registered on http://www.pubmed.gov on the benefits of Cordyceps sinensis, here are a few examples of those trials.

Cordyceps increases cellular oxygen absorption by up to 40% and improves stamina and cellular energy by as much as 55%.

Cordyceps improves the functioning of the heart and helps maintain balanced cholesterol levels.

Cordyceps: Improvement in the reduction of fatigue by 92%, feeling cold by 89%, and dizziness by 83%.

Cordyceps: Chronic kidney disease improvement, improves liver function, improves libido and quality of life in men & women.

RECIPES:

2 MINUTE POWER SMOOTHIE

Breakfast for many is a real rush job. People always seem to be in a hurry in the morning, whether that's because they slept in, are organizing kids for school, or just in a hurry to avoid peak hour traffic, so as to get to work on time.

This is an easy 2-minute breakfast, easy to prepare, balanced, and nutritious. It is rich in protein and will keep you satiated until lunchtime.

INGREDIENTS:

- 2 x Ripe Lady finger bananas
- 2 x Free range eggs
- 1 x Tbsp gelatin powder
- 1 Tbsp Hemp protein powder
- 2 x cups of milk of choice

METHOD:

STEP 1

- Put all the ingredients in a blender and whizz for 1 min until smooth.

STEP 2

- Pour the power smoothie into two glasses and serve.

RECIPES:

POWER PORRIDGE RECIPE

100% organic whole oat groat, power porridge

This is a really wholesome and sustaining breakfast; it is

something you will look forward to each day. Whole oats are a low-energy-dense food and a great warming food which means, they will fill you up and sustain you from one meal to the next and help you avoid snacking between meals. They are the perfect food to start your day, and ideal if you want to lose weight.

WHAT ARE WHOLE OATS OR OAT GROATS

They are the whole oat kernel, with the outer hull removed. Because they have not been rolled or cracked, they retain all their nutritional vitality, unlike rolled oats which start to rancify immediately on rolling, or flaking, and even though stabilizers have been added to the rolled oats, they lose much of their nutritional vitality within 3 days.

That's why whole oat groats will sustain you so much better than rolled oats, they still retain the vitality of all the minerals present in whole oats. Whole oats are high in manganese, and they also contain molybdenum, phosphorus, copper, biotin, vitamin B1, magnesium, fiber, chromium, zinc, and protein, all in balanced proportions the way nature intended them to be.

SLOW COOKER OAT GROAT POWER PORRIDGE INGREDIENTS

SERVINGS: 2 x two cup servings

INGREDIENTS:

- 1 cup whole organic oat groats
- 6 cups of filtered water
- 1 cup of organic sultanas, or raisins, or a combination of both
- 1 teaspoon Celtic sea salt
- 1 cup milk of your choice (dairy or non-dairy)

DIRECTIONS:

- Add 1 cup of organic oat groats to your slow cooker.
- Add 6 cups of filtered water.
- Add 1 cup of organic sultanas, raisins, or a combination of both.
- Add 1 teaspoon of Celtic sea salt.
- Stir the ingredients.

Set the cooker on slow heat for 8 hours before going to bed, so that when you awaken the next morning your breakfast is ready to eat. Or set on high heat for 4 hours during the day.

When cooking time is complete, your organic oat-groat power porridge breakfast is ready to be served.

Add a normal amount of milk of your choice (dairy or non-dairy) and enjoy it.

Refrigerate the remainder for use the next day. Don't be worried if the cooking time slightly exceeds 8 hours, there is sufficient water in the mix, to ensure it doesn't dry out.

For next-day use, you can eat the porridge cold, or slightly warm it by adding a small amount of milk of your choice to the mix and slow cooking it in a saucepan for 5-10 minutes.

The slow cooker is a must in your kitchen, there are many more recipes you can obtain using the slow cooker. As well as cooking the food slowly on regular heat to ensure all the enzymes are not destroyed by heat, helps retain all the juices obtained during the cooking process, so you don't lose any of the goodness from the prepared food.

Why Celtic sea salt? It is the only salt with any scientific validation, that it contains 84 minerals in balanced proportions. It is one of the missing links in cooking, as it adds flavor to the meal and aids in the digestion of the food.

<u>RECIPES:</u>

TOASTIES RECIPE

We have a lot of toasties for meals, and our children love them. They are simple and easy meals to prepare and are very wholesome, tasty, and satisfying.

There are so many variations to toasties, so no one needs ever be bored with their meals.

RECIPES:

SARDINES ON SOURDOUGH TOAST

Sardines are small, oily fish, that are in fact just the younger version of the Pilchard, changing their name once they reach two years old. They are usually fished in the waters around the UK from late June to February when they become widely available. Sardines from around the UK are generally considered to be sustainable fish.

Sardines are not just tasty they are a very healthy food. Sardines are rich in numerous nutrients, in particular, they are a great concentrated source of omega-3 fatty acids and B vitamins which are recognised as being important for heart and brain health. Sardines are also a rich source of bone-building vitamin D.

DIRECTIONS:

Toast the sourdough bread, add butter (optional), add a tin of wild ocean sardines to the bread, and add Celtic sea salt and cracked pepper to taste.

<u>RECIPES:</u>

AVACADOS AND BAKED BEANS ON TOAST

INGREDIENTS:

- 1 x Avacado
- 2 x slices of sourdough bread
- 1 tin of organic baked beans

METHOD:

- Toast bread on both sides
- Spoon over warmed baked beans
- Top each with 1/2 avacado, finely sliced

HAM, TOMATO & CHEESE TOASTIE INGREDIENTS:

- 2 slices sourdough bread
- 2 Tbsp butter
- 2-4 slices of ham to cover the top of the bread
- 1 medium ripe tomato
- 60 grams of Shredded cheddar cheese

INSTRUCTIONS:

- Spread butter on one side of the bread only.
- Place enough ham to cover the top of the bread.
- Thinly slice the tomato to cover the ham.
- Place cheese on top of all ingredients on the bread.
- Place in oven until cheese melts.

RECIPES:
CHICKEN SOUP RECIPE

This chicken soup is easy to make and simply delicious whenever you want to eat something hearty, warm, and comforting.

It is the BEST chicken soup you'll ever eat is the perfect recipe to make when you're feeling sick. Packed with antioxidants like Vitamin A & Vitamin C, that will nourish your body back to recovery.

INGREDIENTS:

- 5 cups of boiling water
- 4 x free-range chicken drumstick pieces
- 3 x slices of ginger
- 3 leaves of lemon grass (tie them in a knot)
- 1 x small white onion
- 1 x spring onion stick
- 1 x bunch of bok choy leaves
- 50 g cabbage
- 1 tsp Celtic sea salt, or to taste
- 1 tsp black pepper

INSTRUCTIONS:

- Place chicken drumsticks, lemon grass and ginger in a boiling pot of water and leave for 30 minutes (until chicken is tender).
- Then add bok choy to the mix for 5 minutes.
- Then add cabbage, salt, and black pepper.
- Leave for 1 minute.
- Done, it is ready to serve with a piece of sourdough bread.
- In season, you can add moringa leaves to the mix.

RECIPES:

FILIPINO PANCIT RECIPE

Pancit is a classic Filipino Recipe. It's a quick and easy stir-fried rice noodle dish with a savory amino sauce, pork and vegetables. My wife is Filipino, she makes this great pancit recipe, and this is one of my favorite meals, along with a slice of sourdough bread and butter.

SERVINGS: 4

INGREDIENTS:

- 100g of pancit Canton, or Chinese noodles
- 2 tablespoons coconut oil
- 200g of chicken strips and 200g of Pork, sliced into bite-size pieces
- 1 brown or white onion diced
- 6 cloves garlic minced
- 3 tablespoons coconut amino sauce, or soy sauce
- 600ml water
- 70g shredded cabbage
- 10 x sticks of green beans sliced
- 60 g capsicum
- 50g broccoli
- 50 g cauliflower
- 2x medium sliced carrots
- 3 x sticks of spring onions (chopped)
- 1x tsp Celtic sea salt and cracked pepper to taste

INSTRUCTIONS:

- In a separate pan, boil water. Put in the noodles and cook, just enough to soften.
- Prep the pork and chicken by cutting them into uniform sizes.
- Heat oil in a wok or large sauté pan. Add pork and chicken and cook for 3-5 minutes until pork and chicken is browned. Set aside on a separate plate.
- Add onion to the pan until soft 1 minute, then add garlic, and mix until brown.
- Add pork and chicken to the mix.
- Add water, amino sauce, salt and black pepper to the pan, and cook for 30-35 minutes, on medium heat, until the pork is tender.
- Add beans, carrots, broccoli, and cauliflower, for 6 minutes (don't overcook).
- Add cabbage and capsicum for 1 minute.
- Remove the pan from the heat.
- Add cooked pancit canton, or Chinese noodles to the mix and stir thoroughly.
- Garnish with spring onions (chopped)
- Serve

RECIPES:

MUNG BEANS & CHICKEN STEW RECIPE

Mung bean & chicken stew is a thick and hearty meal,

especially when eaten with homemade, organic whole-grain sourdough bread. It is an absolutely yummy meal, it is one of my favorites, it is so easy to prepare, it is simple, it satiates you and leaves you with an incredible feeling of satisfaction afterward. It's like you have just eaten a very special meal.

CUSINE: Asian

SERVINGS: 4

INGREDIENTS:

- ½ cup Organic Green Mung Beans (soaked overnight in 2 cups of water to remove phytic acid)
- 400ml water
- 250g free-range chicken strips
- 1 tbsp coconut oil
- 1 small, chopped onion red or white
- 2 garlic cloves, minced
- 15 grams chopped fresh ginger pieces
- ¼ cup light canned coconut cream
- 100 grams of organic or chemical-free cabbage
- 100 grams of organic or chemical-free broccoli
- 100 grams of organic or chemical-free cauliflower
- 50g chemical-free or organic moringa leaves (optional)
- 40 grams of red bell pepper, or Capsicum
- 6g Celtic sea salt (or to taste)
- 1 x yellow onion, minced

INSTRUCTIONS:

- Add 2 cups of water to a pot, add mung beans and soak for 8 hours. After 8 hours, remove excess water from the pot.
- Add 2 cups water to a pot, bring to a boil and add the mung beans.
- Cook the mung beans covered, for about 45 minutes, until the water gets low, and the beans are soft & creamy.
- While your beans are cooking, heat coconut oil in a pot, over medium-high heat and add onion, cook until the onion gets soft (1 minute).
- Add garlic to the mix and cook until garlic gets brown (1 minute).
- Add ginger and stir the mix.
- Add chicken strips and fry for 2 minutes.
- Add 400ml water to the mix and stir, cook for 15-20 minutes, or until chicken is tender.
- Add the creamy mung beans to the mixture and stir. Cover the mixture and it let sit for 1 minute on heat.
- Add, broccoli and moringa to the mix and stir well. Cover the mix and cook for 5 minutes.
- Add capsicum and cabbage cook for 1 minute, then add 6g of coarse Celtic sea salt and black pepper
- Add 1/2 cup of coconut cream to the mix and stir well leave for 1 minute on heat. Your mung bean and chicken stew are ready to eat.
- Serve with 1 slice of homemade organic whole wheat sourdough bread.

SUMMARY

Real bread is the staff of life, it always has been, if the laws of nature are adhered to and bread is baked to biological considerations using a traditional baking process.

Real bread comprising 3 ingredients, whole grain flour, filtered water, and Celtic salt, is more nutritious than any other food, including meat, fruit or vegetables, it will sustain you better than any other food, that's why it needs to become a staple with every meal for the benefit of the health of all people.

This information needs to be passed on to future generations, so they may see and experience the truth behind what makes up real bread. There is so much misinformation about bread and it relates to imposter bread, which is not real bread, rather it is your everyday, white, wholemeal and multigrain bread, an inferior product, masquerading as real bread.

Our young people need to seek the truth, not believe fake news and the proof is always in the eating. Once you bake real bread by traditional means and enjoy its qualities you will know the truth and never return to eating everyday, white, whole meal, or multigrain bread again.

Baking real bread is a true survival skill, knowing how to make real bread means, you will never go hungry and in these times of uncertainty real bread may well be the difference between hunger and having food to eat. Past civilizations were built, sustained and advanced by bread alone and we can return to that healthy way of life, and we may well need to in order to survive, given our world's current situation, regarding the coronavirus.

Whole grain kernels, or berries as we know them, (not ground, rolled, or cut) are all that is required, along with water and Celtic sea salt to make real bread. Sixty kilograms of organic wheat kernels, or more, can be kept with proper storage for 10 years without losing their nutritional value, unlike milled bread flour which stales after 3 days. So real bread-making becomes a pivotal and cost-effective skill for survival.

ABOUT THE AUTHOR

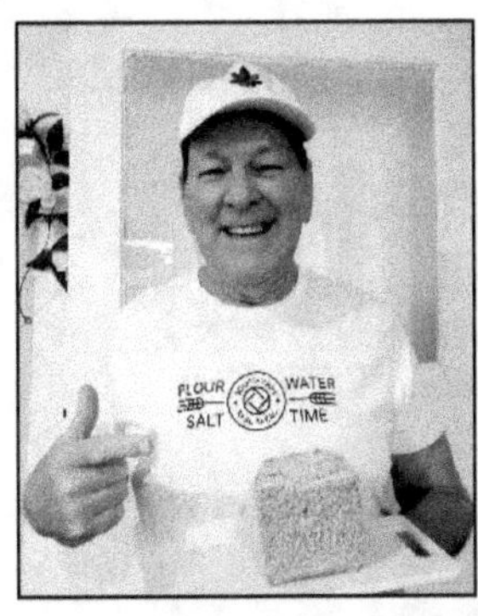

The author of this book, Peter McDonald, is a 3rd generation baker, both his father and grandfather were bakers.

His grandfather Joseph Patrick McDonald opened his first bakery in Mt. Kokeby via Beverley, Western Australia in 1903. A further bakery was opened in Beverley in 1907 and during the depression he and Joseph Peter McDonald (Peter's dad) opened a bakery in the mining town of Mt. Palmer, Western Australia in 1936, right up until the closure of the town in 1942.

Peter has been involved in the health food industry in Australia for over 36 years, as a distributor, teacher, manufacturer, and retailer. He started teaching sourdough bread baking in 1989 using the unique macrobiotic technique perfected by Jacques de Langre of Celtic Sea salt fame. Jacques de Lange (Ph.D. in biochemistry) from Magalia, California, USA, researched and taught the lost art of sourdough bread baking for over 35 years.

Peter has taught the lost art of baking ancestral and allergy-free, sourdough bread, since 1989. In 1994 opened the Celtic Organic Bakery and the Celtic Organic Health Food Store which specialized in whole food, in Alicia St, Southport, Queensland. The Celtic Bakery specialized in providing allergy-free bread and ran for 10 years. A further whole food store was opened at the Pines shopping center, Elanora, Queensland in 2000.

Celtic Organic Bakery was one of a small number of bakeries in Australia, that milled the organic grain on the premises, providing rancid-free sourdough bread to their customers. The organic grain was freshly milled on the premises and used immediately to make rancid-free sourdough bread. The bread was made with 3 ingredients only, Organic flour, filtered water, and Celtic Sea salt, and without the use of processing aids or any other artificial additives. People with wheat and gluten allergies (not celiacs) were amazed at being able to eat real bread without reacting to any existing allergies or intolerance.

Peter still bakes organic, whole wheat sourdough bread for his family and friends and continues to provide advice to people, on how to make real bread.

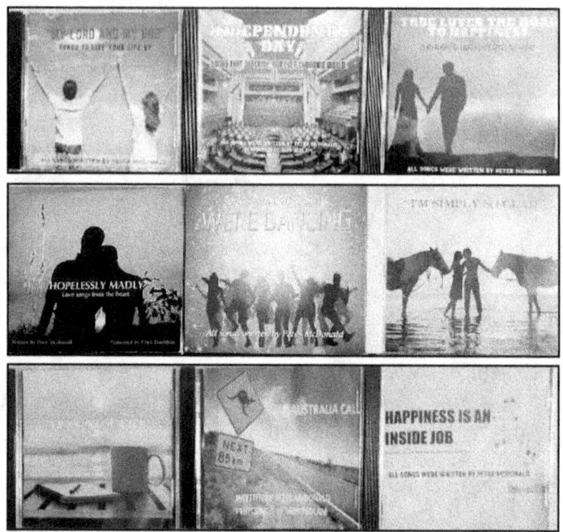

He is a songwriter, his genre is country, folk, pop, protest, and spiritual music, and he has just completed and recorded his ninth album of songs, sung by various artists around the world. He is a scriptwriter and wrote the script and music for the musical "We're Dancing".

His first book " How Cayenne Pepper Saved My Life" is an account of his own amazing recovery from a cardiac arrest using natural remedies.

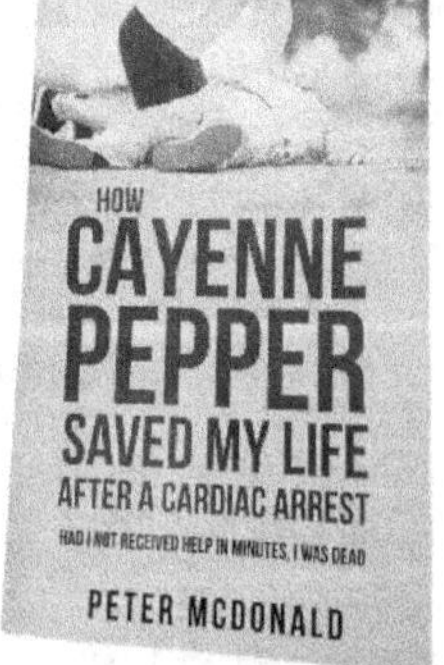

His latest book, "Real Bread, Evil Bread", has been 8 years in the making, and it explains the lost secrets of ancient sourdough and allergy-free bread baking. It is a collation of the notes and information passed on from Jacques de Lange Ph.D. (author of the book "Sea Salts Hidden Powers") and Professor Louis Kervran, (author of the book, "Breads Biological Transmutations) as well as his own information and that of many other great bread bakers of the past.